100 Questions & Answers for Women Living with Cancer

A Practical Guide for Survivorship

Michael L. Krychman, MD
Associate Clinical Attending
Co-Director of the Sexual Medicine Program
Memorial Sloan Kettering Cancer Center
New York, NY

JONES AND BARTLETT PUBLISHERS
Sudbury, Massachusetts
BOSTON   TORONTO   LONDON   SINGAPORE

World Headquarters

Jones and Bartlett
  Publishers
40 Tall Pine Drive
Sudbury, MA 01776
978-443-5000
info@jbpub.com
www.jbpub.com

Jones and Bartlett
  Publishers Canada
6339 Ormindale Way
Mississauga, Ontario L5V 1J2
CANADA

Jones and Bartlett
  Publishers International
Barb House, Barb Mews
London W6 7PA
UK

Jones and Bartlett's books and products are available through most bookstores and online booksellers. To contact Jones and Bartlett Publishers directly, call 800-832-0034, fax 978-443-8000, or visit our website, www.jbpub.com.

Substantial discounts on bulk quantities of Jones and Bartlett's publications are available to corporations, professional associations, and other qualified organizations. For details and specific discount information, contact the special sales department at Jones and Bartlett via the above contact information or send an email to specialsales@jbpub.com.

Library of Congress Cataloging-in-Publication Data
Krychman, Michael L.
  100 questions and answers for women living with cancer : a practical guide for survivorship / Michael L. Krychman.
    p. cm.
  Includes index.
  ISBN-13: 978-0-7637-3924-9
  ISBN-10: 0-7637-3924-3
  1. Cancer in women--Popular works. 2. Cancer in women--Miscellanea. I. Title. II. Title: One hundred questions and answers for women living with cancer.
  RC281.W65K79 2007
  616.99'40082--dc22

                                                                          2006035892

6048

Production Credits
Executive Publisher: Christopher Davis
Associate Editor: Kathy Richardson
Production Director: Amy Rose
Production Editor: Renée Sekerak
Manufacturing Buyer: Therese Connell
Cover Design: Anne Spencer
Composition: Northeast Compositors, Inc.
Cover Image: (clockwise) © Rubberball Productions, © Jessica Bilen/Shutter Stock, Inc., © LiquidLibrary
Printing and Binding: Malloy, Inc.
Cover Printing: Malloy, Inc.

The authors, editor, and publisher have made every effort to provide accurate information. However, they are not responsible for errors, omissions, or for any outcomes related to the use of the contents of this book and take no responsibility for the use of the products described. Treatments and side effects described in this book may not be applicable to all patients; likewise, some patients may require a dose or experience a side effect that is not described herein. The reader should confer with his or her own physician regarding specific treatments and side effects. Drugs and medical devices are discussed that may have limited availability controlled by the Food and Drug Administration (FDA) for use only in a research study or clinical trial. The drug information presented has been derived from reference sources, recently published data, and pharmaceutical research data. Research, clinical practice, and government regulations often change the accepted standard in this field. When consideration is being given to use of any drug in the clinical setting, the healthcare provider or reader is responsible for determining FDA status of the drug, reading the package insert, reviewing prescribing information for the most up-to-date recommendations on dose, precautions, and contraindications, and determining the appropriate usage for the product. This is especially important in the case of drugs that are new or seldom used.

Printed in the United States of America
10 09 08 07 06   10 9 8 7 6 5 4 3 2 1

This book is dedicated to John Franconi and our beautiful twins, Julianna and Russell Franconi-Krychman. You all are my hope, happiness, joy, and the inspiration to my personal success, in life and in my own journey of survivorship. Thank you for your support during the book writing process.

Contents

Questions 1-5 answer most frequently asked questions about cancer survival, such as:

- Who is a cancer survivor?
- Is cancer a chronic illness?
- Now that I have cancer, what do I do?

Questions 6-31 provide information for maintaining good health, including:

- What are age-specific screening protocols?
- Can I increase bone density and strength?
- How can I prevent cancer recurrence?

Questions 32-36 stress the importance of balanced nutrition and diet:

- What are some healthy foods to include in my diet?
- Will taking vitamins help my health?
- How can I use complementary therapies, such as herbs, to help my general health?

Questions 37-41 discuss the need for regular exercise, such as:

- Why should I exercise?
- How do I develop an exercise plan that works for me?
- How can I overcome my resistance to a more active lifestyle?

Questions 42-47 address issues for coping with pain and fatigue, for example:

- What can I do to alleviate my fatigue?
- How is cancer pain treated?
- How can I improve the duration and quality of my sleep patterns?

When colleagues asked me if I was interested in writing a book, I answered quickly that I did have an excellent topic for a patient educational book and would welcome the opportunity to get some of my thoughts down in a book form. As a physician, my clinical practice is twofold: being a gynecologist, I practice survivorship medicine for female cancer patients trying to empower them to make active lifestyle decisions that will promote healthy positive lifestyles; I also am the co-director of the Sexual Medicine and Rehabilitation Program, which focuses on improving sexual functioning for female cancer survivors whose lives are affected by their cancer therapies.

The goals of survivorship medicine include:

- Prevention of disease recurrence
- Prevention of secondary malignancies
- Promotion of general health and recovery
- Lessening and treating the detrimental side effects from primary disease therapy
- Enhancement of global quality of life and relationships
- Empowerment of cancer survivors to make active changes in their lifestyles that improve health and functioning

In 2005 at the age of 36, I was diagnosed with a rare sarcoma. I remember the afternoon clearly as I was on my way to give a lecture on Cancer Survivorship. In the hallway, my surgeon relayed the biopsy results to me: it was positive for cancer. She then informed me that I was going to be all right but that I would need further surgical treatment and even possibly radiation. The shock and echo of cancer began. My world stopped rotating and images of death, disease, pain, and suffering instantly flashed before my eyes. The sadness and shock overwhelmed me as I knew I would have to face parents, family, friends, and loved ones with the burden of cancer.

Next came the treatment phase where surgery was performed twice, and the agonizing wait for pathology, margins status, and final decision of treatment plan. I was fortunate to have the support of my strong significant other and family, who balanced the much needed physical recovery with emotional support and encouragement. While the illness process was going on, I looked at life in a new way. I revised my will, made certain that my affairs were in order, all the while preparing for the worst but hoping for the best. Then without notice, I was told that I was now done with treatment and no more therapy was needed. My surgeon told me to go live and enjoy as I was a "survivor," with the stipulation that I was only considered cured if the cancer did not return within ten years.

I had no tools. I had no survivorship guide or means to begin again after the turmoil of the previous several months. It was not so very long ago that we used to have celebratory parties in the chemotherapy unit once toxic treatments were completed and we told our patients to begin living again. Patients undoubtedly were ill equipped to face the last phase of cancer care—the phase of survivorship or living with cancer.

Whatever words the cancer survivor wishes to use, whether it is cured, in remission, cancer survivor, stabilized disease, or living with cancer, the experience of cancer from diagnosis through treatment and ultimately through your journey of survivorship, I hold fast the belief that, once your life has been touched by the experience of cancer, either with a personal diagnosis or the diagnosis of a close loved one

YOU WILL NEVER BE THE SAME PERSON!

The cancer survivor often needs a moment of freedom from the grip of cancer and its associated thoughts, a break or a needed vacation from cancer. It comes in the form of seconds, then minutes, and then hours followed by days and years. No matter what, there will always be something, some trigger like an advertisement, television commercial, or remark perhaps from strangers, a news program, or a magazine article that will immediately bring the survivor back to that experience of cancer. Perhaps it is that repeat cancer scan, like the MRI you get every six months to watch an area that appears stable and is not growing. Perhaps it is the advertisement concerning an upcoming cancer walk or news heralding a breakthrough treatment for cancer. No matter what it is, something, somewhere, somehow, you will be reminded. Although time lessens the anxiety and emotional charge you may experience with your memories of your horrible time with cancer, unfortunately you will be blessed with the remembrance of this difficult time. Some consider themselves blessed because of the reminder to live strong, being faithful to life's pleasures, all the while embracing the joys, sadness, and beauty of life on a day-to-day basis.

I can only hope that this therapeutic guide, in the form of questions and answers, will help women become empowered so that they may face each day with hope and dignity, and with a strong body, mind, and spirit be active participants in their health care.

I feel privileged for my colleagues at Memorial Sloan-Kettering Cancer Center in the Division of Gynecology–Oncology and General Gynecology.

A special thank you to Dr. Richard Barakat, Chairman of Gynecology–Oncology. I also thank Christina Perkell and Megan Downes for their expertise and skilled nursing care. A special thanks to Carolin Dicembre, who does an excellent job managing the sexual medicine clinic. Thank you, Dr. Mary Sue Brady for your surgical expertise, wisdom, and patience; it's not easy being the surgeon of a surgeon. A particular thanks to Dr. Elizabeth Poynor, who is not only an exceptional career mentor but a close friend. I also thank the medical education staff and nursing department at Memorial Sloan Kettering Cancer Center for their contributions with respect to patient educational materials. I would also like to acknowledge the American Cancer Society and their excellent educational resource materials, which were invaluable in the writing of this book.

Last but not least, I thank Frances Schultz for her contribution and courage. To all the women who battle cancer on a day-to-day basis, who live strong and face adversity with strength, and enthusiasm for survivorship, you are the inspiration for this book. May this help you, the reader, to reclaim your lives after the devastating experience of cancer.

A special acknowledgement goes to my parents, Muriel and Paul Krychman, who with love and encouragement have always showed me that nothing is out of my grasp as long as I am committed to excellence and strive with persistence to achieve my goals. Thank you to my brother and sister-in-law, Steven and Nancy Krychman, and my niece Hailey and nephew Gregory, who have shown me unconditional love and encouragement. To my extended family, Tom and Judy Franconi, and the rest of the Franconi clan, I thank you for your support now and always.

PART 1

Cancer Survivorship

Who is a cancer survivor?

Is cancer a chronic illness?

Now that I have cancer, what do I do?

More...

If we think back, it was not long ago when we used to have celebratory parties in the chemotherapy unit after the patient's completion of the last dose of chemotherapy. We believed that the patients were done. They were finished with their therapy and now they were set to continue living. Only recently has the medical community realized that cancer care is divided into various stages. The *echo stage* is the time when you are sitting in the doctor's office and the physician sitting behind the desk says, "The **biopsy** was positive. It is cancer." Your world stops rotating. The silence is piercing. The world echoes. It vibrates with uncertainty and you feel your stomach contents churn with nausea. You are barely listening and cannot process any more information at this point.

Next you move into the *task phase*, which includes preoperative testing, **CT scans**, **MRI** and **PET scans**, being poked and prodded, needles, intravenous injections, blood tests, and invasion of your personal space. Then begins the *treatment phase*, which often includes surgery, radiation, and/or chemotherapy. You try to get through one experience at a time, just barely keeping your head above water.

Once you are done with your therapies, you are in what most healthcare professionals call the *stage of cancer survivorship*. Perhaps the Lance Armstrong Foundation best defines the term. Cancer survivorship begins at the time of diagnosis. The term *cancer survivor*, according to the Lance Armstrong Foundation, is a person who has been diagnosed with cancer and the people in their lives who are affected by the diagnosis including family members, friends, and caregivers.

Biopsy

a small amount of tissue removed during surgery or a less invasive procedure for later analysis by a pathologist.

Computed tomography (CT scan)

a highly sensitive radiology imaging technique used to help diagnose a disease; used periodically to check the progress of tumors in patients with cancer.

Magnetic resonance imaging (MRI scan)

a diagnostic test that creates images of structures in the body using radio waves and a powerful magnet.

Positron emission tomography (PET scan)

a specialized imaging test used for diagnosis that can see inside sections of the body.

1. Who is a cancer survivor?

According to the Lance Armstrong Foundation executive summary, cancer is the second leading cause of death in the United States and affects an estimated one in three individuals either through their own diagnosis or that of a loved one. Increased technological advancements and medical breakthroughs have led to increased sensitivities of diagnostic tests, and decreased toxicities of treatment have led to improved earlier treatment, and more people surviving cancer.

According to 2003 American Cancer Society statistics, approximately 62% of cancer survivors are expected to live at least five years. As of 2000, there were close to 10 million cancer survivors in the United States but this number does not include others who are directly affected by a malignancy diagnosis like family members, relative's friends, and work colleagues. This estimated number undoubtedly will increase in the years to come.

Cancer patients often do not know what to call themselves. Are they truly survivors, free of disease? Are they living with cancer? Are they cured? In **remission**? Living with advanced disease that is stabilized by medication or chronic **chemotherapy**? No matter what name the cancer survivor calls him- or herself, it is clear they have been irreversibly affected by this illness; they will never be the same person they were before the time of the cancer diagnosis.

2. What is survivorship medicine?

Survivorship medicine includes the general health maintenance of people who have had cancer. Its purpose is to prevent the development of secondary

Remission
subsiding of disease; the disease is still present but either it is undetectable to the patient or it has no symptoms.

Chemotherapy
treatment used after a tumor has been removed surgically to destroy any remaining cancer cells.

cancers whenever possible, and promote health and well being by focusing on primary and preventative care. This encompasses the screening for other cancers.

Survivorship medicine also provides for the support of cancer families, which may include providing resources they need to cope with their illness. Another goal is to minimize pain, disability, and psychosocial stressors while promoting and encouraging improved quality of life. Goals of survivorship medicine encompass prevention and early detection. This involves empowering cancer survivors with the knowledge and tools so that they may make active decisions in how they live their lives. It helps people to live healthy, active, and productive lives even in the face of serious or chronic medical illness.

The Lance Armstrong Foundation refers to living "with" cancer as the experience of receiving a cancer diagnosis and treatment. Living "through" cancer refers to the extended stage following treatment, and living "beyond" cancer refers to the time after treatment, that is, short- and long-term survivorship. Cancer survivors live during and through their illness, but are especially focused and charged with the future. Cancer survivors live through their illness and beyond, no matter the time frame. It could be days, weeks, months, and very often is years. Survivorship is living actively, the best you can so that you enjoy life and have a healthy outlook on the future.

3. Is cancer a chronic illness?

According to the American Cancer Society's *Facts and Figures for 2005*, more than 1.3 million new cases of cancer were expected to be diagnosed in 2005. The National Cancer Institute estimates that approximately 9.8 million Americans with a history of cancer are alive in January 2001. The five-year relative survival rate for all cancers diagnosed between 1995 and 2000 is 64%, which is up from 50% during the years 1974 to 1976. This increased survival rate is due to early detection as well as innovative advances in treatment and supportive care.

Cancer care has become a chronic medical illness not unlike **hypertension** or diabetes. The prevention of treatment side effects and the long lasting effects of treatment are important at the initial stage of diagnosis. Just as an internist will counsel a newly diagnosed diabetic about foot care so that healthy feet hygiene can be maintained, and talk seriously with a newly diagnosed hypertensive woman about diet, salt intake, and exercise regimes to help stabilize her disease, so too is the cancer patient counseled. Cancer may not be cured but may be stabilized. This means that disease is present but does not progress or regress. Women can now live longer, productive, and healthier lives even in the face of advanced or severe metastatic disease. Young children with cancer can now live longer healthy lives, too. Therefore, the issues of improved survivorship and quality of life concerns have gained importance.

Hypertension (also known as high blood pressure)
an abnormally high arterial blood pressure that typically results from a thickening of blood vessel walls; a risk factor for various illnesses such as heart attack, heart failure, stroke, or end-stage renal (kidney) disease.

4. Now that I have cancer, what do I do?

Once they recover from the initial shock of the diagnosis, cancer care becomes focused on, "what I need to do now to get through this." This is typically known as the task phase. It's when you are preoccupied with surgical preparation, radiation, and/or chemotherapy.

But after the initial treatment, most cancer survivors begin to question what else they can do to help decrease their risk for other cancers. This may include a comprehensive physical examination and modification of lifestyle factors that may be destructive to one's physical or emotional health. Others focus on general health maintenance regimes and seek out many healthcare provider specialists to begin intensive screening programs. Others, who want to feel empowered and help maintain good health while minimizing their chances for recurrence, focus on optimum medical health and developing a wellness program/survivorship plan.

Just how does one go about developing such a comprehensive plan? Do you focus on prevention or reducing hazards in your life? Do you become a vegetarian and load up on vitamins and nutritional supplements? Do you search for a sense of spiritual connectedness with your fellow human in the hopes of enriching your mind and strengthening your immunity to ward of illness? Most often the answer is a complex and very personal journey. No two people experience cancer in the same way and no two people will embark on their journey of survivorship in the same fashion. A personalized plan and individual journey is the key to successful survivorship.

As you move further away from your cancer treatment, you may find it difficult to adapt to life again, now as a cancer survivor. You are encouraged that your disease is stabilized or in remission; however, as a survivor, you wish to optimize your health and prevent disease recurrence. Often there is lack of a social network or resources available to help you adjust to cancer survivorship. Resources and organizations that help you transition into life after cancer are listed in the Appendix.

It may sound strange, but from the moment of diagnosis I decided to see this damn cancer as an intended part of my journey in life. Even if I wasn't going to enjoy this part of the trip, I knew there would be lessons for me in it and that it would make me better. Mind you, if anyone else had told me that I would have smacked them, but I could tell myself that and it calmed me. It also gave me confidence and re-confirmed my faith. And while I am happy to call it "my" journey, I almost never say "my" cancer, because it implies an ownership I do not want to claim. I do not intend to keep it, nor do I want to make the cancer feel "welcome" or to "belong" in any way, however subtle or semantic. The smartest doctors in the world still haven't fathomed all the mind does, but we all know it is a powerful thing.

I also decided to go at the cancer with everything I could: I began and stuck to a regular program of meditation and exercise; I consulted a holistic healer; I had a feng-shui practitioner come to my apartment; I prayed; I read inspiring and empowering books by authors such as Wayne Dyer and Marianne Williamson. I rallied my close friends and family and kept quiet about it to everyone else. I didn't want it to be what my life was about. Nor did I want to have to talk about it all the time—or be talked about for that matter. Anything I could do to enhance my environment or frame of mind, I did. Then I went about my life and my work as best I could, as I always had, but I became much more selective about demands on my energy and time. Cancer has a way of reorganizing your priorities, to say the least, and that is a gift.

Frances S.

5. What are some of the common myths of cancer?

Cancer still has many stigmas. When people first learn they have cancer, immediate thoughts of death, pain, and suffering come to mind. However, the face of cancer and the survivor are constantly changing as the medical scientific community makes great strides and advancements on a day-to-day basis. Some of the more common myths of cancer have been adapted from the Lance Armstrong Foundation executive summary and are listed below.

Cancer is a disease that only affects older people.

Close to 80% of all cancers are diagnosed in people over the age of 55. But everyone at any age is at risk for developing a **malignancy**. Young women do get cancer and this is why screening programs are of paramount importance. Many children who once died from pediatric cancers a decade ago are now living to adulthood, enjoying active, healthy lives. Quality of life concerns are critical for them as well.

Cancer only affects those that were diagnosed with the disease.

Many people such as friends, relatives, work partners, and associates are affected either directly or indirectly when someone they know gets cancer. A child diagnosed with cancer dramatically changes the dynamic within the family. A woman who gets breast cancer will affect not only herself but her husband or partner and her children. Roles may become reversed within the family unit. Sometimes the breadwinner must assume many more responsibilities that once had been delegated to another. Extended family members who were less important in the day-to-day management of the household now are critical. Friends and associates may also take on other roles to help the family in crisis.

Cancer is the same for everyone.

The experience of cancer is complex and affects each individual differently. The type, stage, and extent of

Malignant

a type of cancerous tumor that can invade surrounding structures and spread to a distant site in the body; even if treated, malignant tumors may cause death.

disease also influences the course of your illness and your survivorship. There is no set plan or right way to experience your cancer illness, nor is there a correct way to handle all the stress, anxiety, and concerns you may have.

Take the time and allow yourself the opportunity to find your unique path. The journey through cancer and beyond is a difficult path that each cancer survivor must travel in an individual pattern. No two women experience breast cancer in the same way. Each may experience the same side effects and treatment regimes, but how they interpret these changes and adapt to the cancer is a personal journey. Allow yourself the opportunity to plan your own special journey in cancer survivorship.

Diagnosis of cancer means certain death.

Death rates following a cancer diagnosis have steadily decreased over the past several decades. Earlier diagnosis and better treatments have impacted both mortality and morbidity rates for several types of cancers. These facts have changed the face of cancer dramatically over the last several years. We now have less invasive and less aggressive approaches that have increased patient survival. Healthcare providers now realize that we can treat less aggressively so that the patient maintains excellent survival and preserves a high quality of life.

The treatment of breast cancer has progressed from severe mastectomy, where the entire breast tissue is removed, to a simple **lumpectomy**. Surgeons now are performing sentinel lymph node biopsy. Although we give radiation to the entire chest wall, new advances are looking at directed radiation through specific tubing into the site of the individual cancer cells. There

Lumpectomy
excision of a breast tumor with a limited amount of associated tissue.

are also many types of medications that stabilize disease or prevent its growth. In this respect, the cancer is still present but not growing as fast as it would without the medication. Medications may even stop the growth altogether.

With less aggressive treatment strategies, women are still optimizing their survival and gaining the advantage of less disfiguring or harmful treatments. Women with advanced cancer often have the opportunity to prolong their lives, in many instances for extended periods of time. So, planning for survivorship is important for all women regardless of their stage of diagnosis.

PART 2

General Health Maintenance

What are age-specific screening protocols?

Can I increase bone density and strength?

How can I prevent cancer recurrence?

More ...

6. I feel confused about age-specific screening protocols. What are they?

Different organizations and various task forces periodically publish guidelines about when and how people should be screened for a specific disease. For example, the American Cancer Society (ACS), American College of Obstetricians and Gynecologists (ACOG) as well as other associations like the United States Preventative Services Task Force, American College of Cardiology, and American Association of Gastrointestinal Surgeons all produce various age-specific guidelines as to when women should get periodically screened. Many of these guidelines are conflicting. Some indicate that health screening should begin at one age but another states that it is safe to wait until several years later. This can be very confusing.

The bottom line is that your care needs to be tailored to your specific history and your specific medical needs. For instance, women with a strong family history of breast cancer may need annual **mammograms** beginning at the age of 35, but another woman who has had cervical cancer only may need routine, annual screening starting at the age of 50. The confusion is understandable. It is always best to discuss your specific cancer and personal medical history as well as your family history with your healthcare provider. Together, you and your healthcare team can plan a comprehensive, appropriate screening program that is easily followed. Be sure to have a plan where you believe that all of your needs are being met. You should feel comfortable that you are getting all of the appropriate tests at the correct time.

Mammography
a special X-ray imaging of the breast where the radiation exposure of the breast tissue is minimal.

Important facets of the general health screening examinations

According to the American College of Obstetrician and Gynecologists' technical bulletin on primary and preventative care on periodic assessment, some of the important components on a comprehensive physical examination include:

Physical Examination

- Cardiac health (blood pressure, cholesterol screening)
- Pelvic examination (Pap test)
- Dental examinations and X-rays
- Vision examinations
- Diabetes screening with glucose checks
- Medication review of prescribed and over-the-counter medications, herbs and supplements (including vitamins), and prescription medications
- Tobacco, alcohol, and drug use screening
- Breast health and review of breast self-examination (mammography)
- Vaccinations
- Skin screening, sun health and skin cancer prevention

Sexuality Screening

- Contraception
- Review safe sex practices
- HIV and other sexually-transmitted disease screening
- Discussion concerning how to prevent sexually transmitted diseases

Nutrition and Fitness

- Evaluate diet and quantity
- Reinforce portion size and food groups
- Discussion of alcohol
- Review exercise plan and time spent exercising

Psychosocial Evaluation

• Screen for psychiatric illnesses like depression and anxiety
• Evaluation of employment satisfaction and enjoyment
• Rule out job burn out and stress
• Screen for domestic partner abuse (physical, emotional, and sexual)
• Abuse history

Injury Prevention

• Driving record
• Safety belts
• Recreational hazards
• Firearms

Obstetrician

a degreed certified physician specializing in the care of a woman and her offspring during her pregnancy, childbirth, and shortly after her delivery.

Pap test

a type of medical test used for the early detection of cancer, especially of the cervix; involves sampling cells and staining them by a special technique that differentiates diseased tissue from normal tissue; also called *Papanicolaou smear*, *Papanicolaou test*, and *Pap smear*.

Perhaps one of the best references for general health maintenance for women is the American College of Obstetricians' new patient educational pamphlet that has been published recently, entitled *Staying Healthy at All Ages*. This excellent booklet discusses screening, immunizations, and special needs as well as health tips for women of all ages. It can be obtained by contacting your **obstetrician**, gynecologist, or calling the American College directly (see Appendix).

7. What should I know about my general health maintenance?

Your annual health examination is an important aspect of your overall health maintenance. The **Pap test** and cervical cancer screening should occur during each yearly visit to your gynecologist or internist. Pelvic and breast examinations are also very important components as well as discussions concerning smoking cessation and alcohol use. Bone health and **osteoporosis** screening are also very important. Colonic health and prevention of **colon** cancer should also be addressed. If you are still having your menstrual cycles, contraception should be reviewed. Safe sex education, sexually transmitted infection protection, and the proper use of latex condoms and lubricants should be reviewed also.

Some tests that may be done are blood pressure measurements, height and weight, and other vital signs. Monitoring your height and weight can be helpful with balancing nutrition and exercise regimes. Periodically, you should also have your cholesterol and lipid profiles checked. Lipid profiles should be done every five years starting when you reach age 45. A thyroid stimulating hormone test should be done annually starting at age 50, and you should have an annual immunization for influenza. Some women may also qualify for certain specific cancer screening programs like ovarian cancer screening. This can be incorporated into your annual visit to your healthcare provider.

8. What is heart health? How can I control my blood pressure?

What was once thought to be a "man's disease" is actually a significant health concern for women. Heart disease is estimated to be the number one killer for women, claiming up to 500,000 lives per year in the United States. Annually, more women actually die from cardiovascular diseases than from all types of cancer combined.

Diseases that affect the arteries, veins, and other blood vessels are often grouped together as cardiovascular

Osteoporosis
a condition that is characterized by a decrease in bone mass and density (thinning of the bones), causing bones to become fragile.

Colon
the large intestine, which is part of your gastrointestinal tract. Its function is to absorb water and food and to excrete stool.

General Health Maintenance

disease. Some of these diseases include: angina (where the heart does not get enough blood which can lead to crushing chest pain); atherosclerosis (narrowing of the arteries with fatty deposits and plaques, which can build up and cause narrowing of the blood supply to the heart, leading to a heart attack or myocardial infarction); coronary heart disease; and heart failure or stroke. Some risk factors for heart disease in women include: diabetes, smoking, hypercholesterolemia, obesity, age, ethnicity, and family history.

Hypertension (high blood pressure) is also another risk factor for developing cardiac disease. The woman who is overweight, not physically active, who smokes cigarettes, and drinks alcohol is typically more at risk for hypertension. Elevated blood pressure is often called the *silent killer*, because often you have no symptoms that signal the disease. A woman may have significant heart damage and disease without even knowing it. Sudden death cardiovascular events, heart attacks, and other forms of heart disease do happen in women without warning. High blood pressure typically occurs in women over the age of 40 and is more common in African-American women. Hypertension commonly runs in families so there may be a genetic component. Knowing your family history is always important, so tell your doctor if your mother or father has hypertension. Certain medical illnesses like diabetes and kidney disorders can be linked to high blood pressure.

Your blood pressure can easily be measured during your annual visit with your gynecologist or internist. If your doctor finds that you have high blood pressure, there are many interventions that can be done before you must start medications. Some lifestyle modifications can help lower your blood pressure and therefore your risks for adverse cardiac events. Weight reduction and maintaining an appropriate body weight; increasing your daily exercise; diet modification with reduced **caffeine**, sodium, and saturated fats intake; stopping smoking; and decreasing your alcohol consumption are among the effective lifestyle modifications that you can put in place to help control blood pressure.

Healthcare professionals encourage all patients to implement weight reduction strategies and maintain an ideal body mass close to 25. You can easily calculate your body mass index (BMI) by the following formula:

Weight in kilograms ÷ Height in meters squared

You also can figure out your BMI using weight in pounds and height in feet and inches by using several Web sites on the Internet. Just search for the key phrase, *calculate body mass index* and several choices will appear on your computer's screen.

Diets high in fruits, vegetables, and fiber with low quantities in saturated fats appear to be heart healthy. Questions 32 through 36 contain helpful suggestions and easy changes that you can make to improve your diet today.

Sometimes conservative lifestyle changes fail to control hypertension. In these cases, medications are needed to control the high blood pressure. Be sure to consult with your physician concerning the type, class, and amount (dose) of medications you may be required to take. It is critical that you take your medications on a regular basis when prescribed even if you have no symptoms. It is important to remember that specific chemotherapy agents may have had some impact on

Caffeine

a naturally occurring substance found in coffee and tea, most soft drinks (sodas), and many energy drinks. This substance can be added to medications for headaches. It acts as a nervous system stimulant and can increase mental alertness and wakefulness.

your heart and might contribute to congestive heart failure. Thus, it is always advisable to ask your oncologist if you should be particularly concerned about long-lasting cardiovascular system (heart) effects from your specific regime and dosing of chemotherapy.

Maintaining a healthy blood pressure is one of many facets for healthy heart care. You should maintain a balanced weight, have your cholesterol checked and monitored, and not smoke; you also should enjoy an active exercise regime. Some of the more advanced screening tests for cardiovascular health include an electrocardiogram or an exercise stress test. You may be a candidate for these tests. If so, they are easy, painless tests that will give your **cardiologist** a lot of useful information concerning your heart health.

Cardiologist

a degreed and certified physician who specializes in the study of the heart and its action and diseases.

9. What is osteoporosis? Why is bone health important?

Osteoporosis is a significant medical illness that affects both men and women as they age. Bone loss can lead to chronic back pain, pain when you are walking, deformity of the bones or spine, and the **dowager's hump**. It is also a risk factor for fracturing a bone in the event of a fall. More than an estimated million fractures in the United States can be attributed to osteoporosis.

Dowager's hump

an abnormal outward curvature of the upper back; round shoulders and spinal changes result in an abnormally stooped posture. This can be caused especially by bone loss and compression of the vertebrae, which commonly occurs in osteoporosis.

The primary goal for managing and treating menopausal osteopenia (slight bone loss below the expected norm for your age group) or osteoporosis is to prevent fractures. With the loss of hormones and with natural aging, your bones can lose their density and become thin, weak, and fragile. Other risks for lowered bone mass density include a previous fracture, your gender (women are more likely than men to have lowered bone density), your age (older women are at a greater risk), and genetics (you are at a greater risk for osteoporosis if your mother or grandmother had osteoporosis). Diets that are low in calcium, extreme thinness, chronic medical conditions like rheumatoid arthritis, thyroid dysfunction, kidney and liver disease as well as some gastrointestinal disorders, a sedentary (non-active) lifestyle, smoking, and excessive alcohol consumption are also considered risk factors.

If you are taking medications like steroids, mediations for thyroid function or some **anticoagulants** (blood thinners) or anti-seizure medications, these may influence your bone strength. Some breast cancer survivors take a class of medications called *aromatase inhibitors*, which include Femara®, Arimidex®, or Aromasin®. These medications may contribute to bone loss, so if you are taking an aromatase inhibitor, you may need to have frequent bone density tests. These medications can often interfere with estrogen production, which is a critical hormone for bone metabolism and health.

Anticoagulant
a type of medication or substance (as a drug) that slows or stops fluid from clumping, especially coagulation of the blood. Also known as a blood thinner.

In the United States, it is estimated that at least 30% of men and women over age 60 will experience a fall at least one time per year. The morbidity and mortality from a fall that results in a fracture are astronomical. Some women with severe osteoporosis even can experience a spontaneous bone break without a significant trauma. Approximately 25% of hip fracture victims over the age of 50 die within one year of the fracture. It is also estimated that up to one third of the remainder will become permanent residents of nursing homes. Many do not regain independent living. Osteoporosis and broken bones associated with poor bone health are a major health concern and have significant ramifications on your lifestyle and quality of life.

Bone density testing involves a dual energy X-ray absorptionmetry (DEXA scan) or bone densitometry. These are painless tests that assess the bone quality in the spinal column, femur (long bone in the thigh), and sometimes wrist and ankle bones. Women usually take this test every two years after the time when they have gone into natural or surgically- or chemically-induced menopause. Under certain conditions when you are taking special medications, like breast cancer survivors who are taking aromatase inhibitors, you may need to get this bone test more often. The results of this test will help your physician manage your bone health more effectively.

How do I prevent falls?

Part of the comprehensive management for osteoporosis includes not only bone health but also an assessment and educational program to help women reduce their potential for falls. Women should be evaluated by their healthcare provider concerning loss of consciousness, fainting, muscle weakness, dizziness, and even for balance problems. Vision and arthritis are also medical conditions that need appropriate assessment and treatment so that good balance can be maintained, which will help prevent falls. You should have your vision checked on an annual basis and replace old glasses as your prescription changes. All types of prescription medications that can possibly affect level of consciousness, balance, and gait should also be re-evaluated on a regular basis.

Safe and sturdy footwear should replace high spiked heeled shoes. Comfort and safety should take priority over style and fashion. Those who are frequent night-time risers should keep the area around their bed clear of objects such as shoes or slippers. Strategically placed nightlights are helpful for nighttime risers. Safety hazards in the home are also a concern. Rug fringes, poor lighting, and cluttered furniture all contribute to falls. Walkways should be clutter-free. Electric and phone wires or extension cords should be tidy and secured to walls, as they can be falling hazards. Grab bars in showers and no skid mats in bathtubs are also essential to help prevent loss of balance and falls.

It is also important to pay close attention when out and about in the street walking or doing outdoor tasks. Inevitably, falls happen when the woman is multitasking, like chatting on her cell phone while walking fast through a crowd, or reading a book while trying to answer her blackberry, or hailing a cab while trying to control small children. So it is important to pay close attention to your surroundings. This is especially important during inclement weather. Rain makes surfaces slippery, snow storms may decrease visibility, and icy patches may be treacherous footing that lead to falls.

10. What can I do to maintain a good bone density and prevent further bone loss?

Calcium and exercise are the mainstays for bone preservation. A calcium supplement may help you to maintain bone strength. It is always best to consult with your healthcare provider to discuss how much (dosage) and how often you should be taking calcium. It is important to know that the body can only absorb a certain amount of calcium at a time, so combining your multivitamin with a calcium supplement may not be the best way to take both of these supplements. It is also important to know that calcium has the potential to interfere with other medications you may also be taking. It's always advisable to consult with your healthcare provider when thinking about adding calcium to your diet.

A recent study from Rabin Medical Center in Israel showed that people who have a colonic polyp (a small growth of tissue that may be a precursor to cancer) and take calcium may have a 26% lower risk for the development of subsequent polyps. Although this evidence does not support the use of calcium to prevent colorectal polyps or cancer, the results are interesting and provocative. Not all patients can tolerate calcium, especially at high doses, and many may suffer from cramps or constipation with these supplements.

There are ongoing and heated debates about the usefulness of calcium supplementation. Controversy appears both in the medical journals and the media. Researchers are now questioning whether calcium supplementation is actually beneficial to overall bone health and maintenance. How much of the calcium do you actually need? How much does the body absorb? Does calcium really impact bone health? Until the dust settles, it seems prudent to enjoy a well balanced diet that is rich in a variety of healthy foods, including nutrients like calcium. It may be wise to have some type of minimal calcium supplementation.

Medications to prevent bone loss

If increased exercise and calcium intake does not maintain (stabilize) your bone loss, your healthcare provider may suggest a medication in the class called *bisphos-*

phonates. The most commonly prescribed medications are risedronate (Actonel®) and alendronate (Fosomax®). Both these medications need to be taken on an empty stomach, with the person sitting upright for at least one half hour; the dose can be on a once a week schedule. The most common side effects are upper gastrointestinal upset and irritation. A newer medication on the market is ibandronate sodium (Boniva®), which has a one tablet per month dose. Although a once monthly dosing sounds very attractive, it is not always the best choice for you and your bones. All of these medications can reduce the bone breakdown that can occur during the transition from having a monthly menstrual cycle to menopause. Research has shown that both Actonel® and Boniva® reduce the risks of spinal (vertebral) fractures at three years in postmenopausal osteoporosis. Actonel® reduces non-vertebral fractures, including the hip, wrist, pelvis, femur, forearm, and collarbone (clavicle).

It is always best to ask your healthcare specialist and bone physician about which medication is the best choice for you. Some patients who take biphosphonates complain of bone and joint pain. The widely publicized medical concern of *osteonecrosis* of the jaw is a rare occurrence that has been reported in some patients receiving biphosphonates. Osteonecrosis is where the blood supply to the bone is interrupted (temporarily or permanently), which causes the bone tissue to die and—if untreated—the bone may collapse. Most cases occur in patients who had cancer and underwent dental procedures; most of them were receiving intravenous types of medications.

Some women may be taking a new medication called raloxifene hydrochloride (Evista®), which is a selective estrogen receptor modulator (SERM) for bone health. Exciting preliminary medical research has shown that Evista® may be helpful in the prevention of breast cancer.

Calcitonin (miacalcin injection, Calcimar®) is another medication that can be prescribed to women who cannot tolerate the biphosphonates. It is a hormone that is produced from the thyroid gland and it can help maintain bone density. Currently used as a nasal spray, calcitonin is known to be less effective than other agents and has not been shown to prevent hip fractures. Raloxifene and tamoxifen are both SERMs that can help preserve bone (see Question 17). These are synthetic hormones that can mimic the action of estrogen in bone tissue, but their side effects can be concerning. Both medications can increase the intensity and number of hot flashes and may cause life-threatening blood clots. Teriparatide (Forteo®) is a daily injectable medication that can promote new bone growth and has been shown to improve bone density in some women.

Pedometer

a small device that can measure your steps, calories burned, and distance that you have walked or jogged.

Exercise, especially weight-bearing activities like walking, jogging, walking up stairs, or climbing, have been proven to maintain bone health. Even activities like dancing and weight training can help with bone preservation. A **pedometer** is a small device that can be purchased from your local sporting goods store to measure the total number of steps you walk each day. It can also measure calories burned and the distance you have traveled. Many women find these small devices very helpful when trying to maintain an active exercise plan. By wearing this small pedometer, you are more aware of the type and amount of your exercise, and so can make conscious decisions to increase your activity. Some women may take the longer route home, skip the taxi and walk the extra few blocks, or forgo the escalator and walk up several flights of stairs. All of these are small things you can do on a daily basis to help you attain some bone health and improve your feelings of general well being.

CANCER PREVENTION

11. What is the Pap test for cervical cancer? How often do I need it?

The Pap test (named for its developer, George Papanicolaou) is the most accurate method to detect cervical cell abnormality at an early stage. This is important so that the abnormal cells can be treated before they may develop into a more serious condition or even cancer. Since its introduction in the United States, the Pap test has lowered the number of deaths from cervical cancer by a dramatic 70%. The Pap test (also called Pap smear) can help you prevent cancer from the cervix.

Located at the mouth of the uterus, the cervix opens into the vagina. It dilates during childbirth to allow the fetus to pass from the uterus into the vagina and finally into the world. The cells of the cervix are constantly growing and shedding. Your physician makes a tiny scrape of these surface cells and analyzes them to see if any abnormality exists.

The Pap smear should be an important part of your annual visit with your internist or obstetrician/gynecologist. Generally, your first Pap test should occur at the age of 21 or shortly after you become sexually active. But the American Cancer Society, the American Association of Colposcopy and Cervical Pathology, and the American Society of Obstetricians and Gynecologists have varying guidelines as to the frequency you should have this test performed. According to the American College of Obstetricians and Gynecologists, it is always wise to consult with your healthcare provider and make a management plan together as to the frequency of Pap smears. If you have had three consecutive Pap tests that are normal and you are over the age of 35, you may be a candidate to have a Paps less frequently than during your annual exam. Also, if you have had a **total hysterectomy** where the cervix has been removed for non-cancerous (**benign**) reasons, you may also not need a Pap done on a yearly basis. Of course, past history and other important medical issues must be taken into consideration. Discuss it with your healthcare provider at your next annual visit.

If you have some of the risk factors for cervical cell abnormalities, you may still need annual Pap smears. Some of the concerning risk factors include: early age of intercourse, intercourse with multiple partners or having partners that have multiple partners, smoking cigarettes, having certain sexually transmitted diseases like human papilloma virus, having a weakened immune system from human immunodeficiency virus (HIV), undergoing chemotherapy, or bone marrow transplantation. Even if you and your doctor have decided that you are not going to get Pap smears on an annual basis, it is still important to visit the doctor on a yearly schedule so that your healthcare provider can examine the vulvar and vaginal tissues as

Total hysterectomy

surgical removal of the uterus and cervix.

Benign

a type of non-cancerous tumor that can grow and press on surrounding structures, but does not invade surrounding structures or spread to a distant site.

well as perform a pelvic examination and a comprehensive medical evaluation.

Abnormal cervical cells may progress from differing grades from minor, mild abnormalities to more moderate cell changes before they become cancer. It is always best to have the Pap smear when you are not menstruating (having your period), and you should not douche or use vaginal medications or spermicide several days before the test.

The Pap test is quite simple, actually. An instrument called a speculum is inserted into the vagina so your clinician can see the cervix. Using a small brush, spatula, or broom-type tool, the cervical cells are collected and placed onto a glass slide. Most institutions are now using a liquid-based Pap test, the most popular of which is called the Thin Prep®.

After it is completed, the cell sample is sent to a laboratory. There the cells are made into a microscope slide that is examined by a computer as well as a trained cytopathologist (a specially trained physician expert in disease changes in cells). A technologist will examine the cells and then classify them as normal or abnormal. Most insurance plans will cover the cost of your annual Pap smear examination.

According to the National Cancer Institute, the Pap smear results can be classified into several categories.

- NORMAL is when only normal cervical cells are visualized.
- ASCUS (atypical cells of undetermined significance) is when there are minor changes seen in the

outer layer of the cervical cells. You may need a colposcopy (see below) or earlier repeat Pap smear.

- SQUAMOUS INTRAEPITHELIAL LESIONS are abnormalities in cervical cells that are classified as either low or high grade. Low grade changes can be associated with the human papilloma virus and are often considered mild changes. In many young women, these types of cells may repair themselves.

Often, with continued surveillance and close follow-up, your Pap tests can return to normal. Close follow-up and patient **compliance** are needed in these cases. About 60% of younger women with low-grade squamous intraepithelial lesions (LGSIL) will have their tests revert back to being normal if they are repeated within six months. High-grade lesions (HGSIL) are more troublesome and many consider them to be precancerous cell changes that warrant further therapy. Most likely, if your Pap smear shows these high grade types of cells, you will require additional testing that may include a colposcopy (discussed below) and biopsies.

Atypical glandular cells of undetermined significance (AGUS) are when the cells that are glands show some abnormalities. When your smear shows this cell type, you may need more testing, including an endometrial biopsy.

Fast facts about the human papilloma virus (HPV)
- Over 100 types of viruses can affect women.
- Only about 30 of these types are sexually transmitted and cause genital HPV.
- Genital HPV can be spread from skin to skin contact and not through the exchange of bodily fluids.
- Genital HPV cannot be prevented by condom use.

Compliance

the process of following a regimen of treatment; the act of taking and following prescribed medications and or instructions given by your healthcare provider.

- The virus is often asymptomatic, which means you may be infected and not show any symptoms.
- About 5.5 million new genital HPV cases occur each year.
- About 20 million men and women are thought to have active HPV infections.
- Nearly three quarters of all Americans between the ages of 15 and 49 have been infected with genital HPV in their lifetime.
- HPV can be contracted from one partner and remain dormant, only later to be unknowingly transmitted to another sexual partner including a spouse.
- Though usually harmless, some subtypes (HPV 16, 18, 31, and 45) are associated with nearly all cases of squamous cell carcinoma of the cervix.
- The best way to screen for cervical cancer is through the Pap test, which may be done alone or in combination with an HPV DNA test.

What is a colposcopy?

If the results of your Pap smear show abnormal cells, your healthcare provider probably will ask you to repeat the Pap test in several months or ask you to undergo additional testing, such as a **colposcopy**. During the colposcopy, a machine called the *colposcope*, which is a binocular-like machine that magnifies the view up to 60 times, is used to look at the details of the cervix. A speculum examination is done (see Question 11) and then the cervix is cleansed with a vinegar (acetic acid) solution to enhance some of the specific features of the cervical cells. Next, the colposcope is used to look at the cervical tissue under various magnifications. Sometimes a special green flitered light is used so that the clinician can see blood vessels better.

Colposcopy

a procedure that uses a specialized machine called a colposcope, which is a magnifying instrument designed to facilitate visual inspection of the vagina and cervix. Women with abnormal cells on their Pap test may be required to undergo this outpatient procedure to visualize and possibly sample (biopsy) the cervical tissues.

If your doctor sees some abnormalities in the cervical tissues, which can include color changes, new blood vessels, or a cobblestone appearance, then a biopsy may be preformed. A *biopsy* is usually a quick procedure where a tiny bit of tissue is removed. You may feel some pinching, burning, pelvic pain, and discomfort during the biopsy, but it usually subsides after a few minutes. The bleeding can be stopped with any one of a variety of different agents, but most often with either silver nitrate or another substance called mons cells. Silver nitrate or mons cells can be applied to the biopsy site to stop bleeding. These agents can sometimes cause abnormally colored discharge. It is important to ask the doctor who preformed your biopsies about specific instructions of what you should do after the colposcopy. Most advocate no heavy lifting, nothing in the vagina, no sexual intercourse for a period of time, no douching, and to call if you experience severe bleeding, pain, fever, or foul smelling discharge from the vagina. Depending on the biopsy results, you may need further therapy or perhaps just close follow-up with repeat Pap smears every few months.

The most important thing to remember is that the vast majority of women who have abnormal cells do not have cervical cancer. If the cells are abnormal and found early, simple procedures can be done to treat these conditions.

Do preventative cervical cancer vaccines exist?

A new vaccine (called Gardasil®, manufactured by Merck Pharmaceuticals) has been shown to protect women against the most common strains of the human papilloma virus (HPV; see Question 11), a virus that can cause cervical cancer. The vaccine is very effective in preventing cervical cancer and genital warts. It is a quadravalent vaccine (meaning it is active against four strains: HPV 6, 11, 16, and 18) and is presently on the market. This vaccine, which consists of 3 shots given over a period of time, is now available for girls and women between the ages of 9–26 and should be given before the beginning of sexual activity. Consult your healthcare provider for more specific medical information. Another pharmaceutical company (GlaxoSmith Klein, manufactures Cervarix®) has developed a bivalent vaccine (active against two strains: HPV 16 and 18) and it is also expected to be available sometime in 2007. Studies of both vaccines have shown that they protect against the human papilloma virus for up to two years so booster shots may be needed. If you may be a candidate for the vaccine, it's best to discuss it with your healthcare provider.

Both vaccines are being considered for young women before they have engaged in sexual activity and are not infected with HPV. However, who in fact is an appropriate candidate remains to be determined. Because many women who are already sexually active may want to be immunized, many will seek out information from their healthcare provider concerning vaccination.

It is important to know that, even with the advent of a cervical vaccine, cervical cancer is not a thing of the past. Most women still need to have annual Pap smears and so must visit their obstetricians and gynecologists on a regular basis for cervical screening. Some important questions remain unanswered. Exactly how long does the immunity last? Does the vaccination provide a decade of protection or does its effectiveness wax and wane over time, thus requiring repeated booster shots? Are the medical community and their female patients able to comply with a strict vaccination schedule? Although the medical community can anticipate that there will be fewer Pap smears (requiring fewer colposcopies and surgical interventions), cervical screening undoubtedly will continue. If you have been one of the first women to receive this vaccination, consult with your healthcare provider about your screening timetable and schedule.

12. Is there a screening for uterine cancer? What is an endometrial biopsy?

Cancer of the uterus is a common female reproductive pelvic **tumor** that is often associated with abnormal vaginal bleeding. Some of the risk factors for developing uterine cancer include: obesity, unopposed **estrogen** use (estrogen without the addition of a progesterone agent when you have a uterus), a positive family history for breast, ovarian or uterine cancer, early **menstruation**, and late **menopause**. The use of the drug tamoxifen in breast cancer patients (see Question 17) also increases the risk of uterine cancer. If your menstrual periods started early or finished later in life, or you have had polycystic ovarian syndrome, or never had a child, then you also may be at an increased risk for developing uterine cancer. According to the American Cancer Society, other risk factors may include infertility and hereditary nonpolyposis colon cancer. Risk of uterine cancer is reduced with pregnancy and the use of combined oral contraceptive pills.

Although there is no screening test for uterine cancer, women who experience any type abnormal vaginal

Tumor

a mass of cells or tissue that grows abnormally.

Estrogen

a female hormone produced by the ovaries; it is responsible for female changes during maturity.

Menstruation

vaginal bleeding due to endometrial shedding following ovulation when the egg is not fertilized.

Menopause

physical changes marking the end of a woman's fertile years, the most notable being the cessation of the menstrual cycles.

bleeding and who are of risk should consult their healthcare provider immediately. They may need an appropriate evaluation that could include an endometrial biopsy and a transvaginal ultrasound (see Question 14), which will look at the endometrium or the uterine lining as well as the pelvic and genital anatomy.

An **endometrial biopsy** is sometimes necessary if you have an abnormal Pap (AGUS) or if you are over age 35 and have abnormal vaginal bleeding. This test is done during the speculum examination, where a small catheter is placed within the uterine cavity and a sample of uterine tissue is taken and sent to the laboratory for analysis. The biopsy can tell if there is an abnormality in the endometrial tissues.

Endometrial biopsy
an office-based procedure where a small plastic instrument called a pipelle is placed within the uterus and a small sample of uterine or endometrial tissue is obtained.

If you are a breast cancer survivor who is on tamoxifen and experience any type of abnormal vaginal bleeding, then you may also need an endometrial biopsy. Tamoxifen acts as an antagonist in the breast, that is, it stops the growth of tissue and prevents further growth. However, it may promote endometrial lining growth. This abnormal growth can lead to the development of endometrial polyps or an endometrial pathology called *hyperplasia* (when the increased number of normal cells actually adds size to the organ). In rare cases, it can lead to endometrial cancer. Because tamoxifen may be associated with endometrial problems, it is very important to tell your breast doctors if you have experienced any abnormal vaginal bleeding. Your gynecological evaluation may include a transvaginal ultrasound or an endometrial biopsy to rule out any underlying abnormality within the uterus. Sometimes a polyp is found that can be removed by a simple outpatient surgical procedure.

General Health Maintenance

13. How can I prevent vulvar cancer?

The vulva is considered the outer part of the female reproductive tract and sometimes is called the lips of the vagina. Cancer of the vulva and clitoris are rare; however, early diagnosis and treatment are needed to prevent spread of the disease. Smoking, HPV infection, multiple sexual partners, HIV infection, or a history of cervical abnormalities may all contribute to the development of vulvar cancer.

Because there is no recommended screening test to detect vulvar or clitoral cancer, it is important to note if you have any unusual symptoms including itchiness, burning in the vulvar area, dry scaly skin changes, bleeding, or abnormal discharge from the vulvar area. You should report these changes to your doctor. Often your doctor may perform a small outpatient biopsy, which is needed to get a definitive diagnosis of the troubling area. It is always wise to examine your vulvar area with the aid of a hand-held mirror and report any changes in skin color or changes in surface texture to the doctor. Many women in fact do have some moles or hemangiomas (an abnormally dense collection of small blood vessels called capillaries) in the vulvar region that can be monitored over time. If they change in characteristics, it is important to report any differences to your gynecologist. Remember that vulvar cancer does have a high cure rate if it is discovered and treated early.

14. What is ovarian cancer screening?

Nearly 25,000 women are diagnosed with ovarian cancer in the United States every year, but unfortunately, there may not be any early symptoms or signs that help physicians diagnose this disease at an early stage. The most common symptom for ovarian cancer in its advanced stages is the accumulation of abdominal fluid and subsequent abdominal enlargement. Sometimes women complain of vague increased abdominal bloating, gas, or stomach discomfort. Ovarian cancer does not have any specific, clear cut presenting symptoms. Very often, patients present with disease that is advanced in stage and has spread to many pelvic or abdominal organs. Some of the vague symptoms associated with ovarian cancer may be abdominal gas or unexplained bloating that does not go away, pelvic pressure, or a swollen abdomen. Recent research indicates that some women complain of urinary symptoms in the early stages of ovarian cancer.

The incidence of ovarian cancer increases with age and the highest risk is after a woman reaches age 70. Those women who are at an increased risk for developing the disease and have a greater than normal chance of getting the cancer at a younger age than the general population may gain some benefit from ovarian cancer screening. This increased risk population includes: women with a known genetic mutation for ovarian cancer; no personal cancer history but a strong family history for either breast or ovarian cancer; or a personal history of breast cancer before the age of 50. Some ethnic groups like women of Ashkenazi Jewish descent and those with a family history of certain cancers may also be at an increased risk. Other factors that may slightly increase your risk for ovarian cancer include: being postmenopausal, overweight, starting to menstruate early and going through menopause later in life, not having any children, history of infertility, or even perhaps the use of talcum powder (see Question 26) on the genital area, especially if the powder contains asbestos as it did over twenty years ago. Being at an increased risk for the disease does not mean you will definitely get the disease, but you may benefit from a screening program. Pregnancy, having a **tubal ligation** (also known as having your tubes tied, which is a form of permanent sterilization), or the use of oral contraceptive pills may in fact reduce your risk for getting ovarian cancer.

Screening for ovarian cancer is not presently medically recommended for the average woman whose risk is not increased.

For those who are at high risk, screening tests may include a **transvaginal ultrasound** to assess the ovaries, regular pelvic examinations, and blood testing to measure CA125 (*c*ancer *a*ntigen 125, which measures a sugar protein that increases when tissues are inflamed or damaged). Many cancer institutions have functionalized screening programs so you can have a regular visit scheduled every six months with your healthcare provider, and some may include a genetic evaluation with a counselor or a genetic specialist.

A transvaginal ultrasound is a specialized ultrasound scan that uses sound waves to image different internal organs. A probe fits within the vagina to better look at the ovaries and the other pelvic organs, and sometimes cysts. It is important to note that ovarian cancer screening is only recommended for those at higher risk for developing ovarian cancer. The test is not 100% specific and sensitive, which means that while the test may show abnormalities, it does not mean that you have cancer. Ovarian cancer screening testing can

Tubal ligation

the destruction or ligation (tying) of the fallopian tubes to prevent passage of the egg or ova from the ovaries into the uterus; a method of female sterilization or contraception.

Transvaginal ultrasound

an imaging technique using high frequency sound waves; a probe is placed in the vagina to assess the female pelvic anatomy.

cause a lot of anxiety for the patient because very often the scan finds harmless simple pelvic cysts that lead to additional ultrasound tests and further evaluations. It may also lead to an unecessary surgery that fails to discover any abnormality or cancer. Presently, many institutions are conducting sophisticated research into specific proteins in the blood that might be useful in diagnosing ovarian cancer in its early stages. These tests are still considered experimental and are not available for the general population.

15. Explain genetic testing and counseling. Why might I need them?

Some cancers run in families. If you had cancer at a young age or have multiple relatives within your immediate family who have had cancer, then you may be interested in getting genetic counseling. If someone in your family has been diagnosed with bilateral (meaning both sided) cancer in paired organs like ovaries, breasts, or kidneys, if more than one blood relative has the same type of cancer, or your relative has an inherited cancer gene, then you also may qualify for genetic testing.

Genetic counseling involves the discussion of your personal and family's risk for the development of certain types of cancers. Because many cancers can be inherited through genes, many people in the same family have the same type of disease. These are called *cluster families*. For example, breast, ovarian, colon, and uterine cancers are prevalent in certain families. Specialized counselors will discuss your specific family history. Then the experts construct a family tree (called a *pedigree*) with the cancers noted on the diagram, and use it to calculate your specific risk to develop other cancers. This testing and analysis can be helpful for you and your relatives. A typical visit lasts one to two hours with the discussion ranging from your risk factors to recommendations for cancer prevention. They may suggest certain recommended screening protocols. Genetic testing typically involves blood laboratory testing to determine if certain genes or blood markers are present. The presence or absence of the specific genes in question can help you plan your medical treatment whether it is for future screening or risk-reducing prophylactic surgery.

One of the most important issues to remember is that when attending the genetics visits, neither you nor your family members are mandated to take the blood test. This meeting is an opportunity for education. Educating yourself and your family about your future cancer risks is an important part of your overall survivorship plan and will factor into your personal screening protocol.

Confidentiality of test results. Most specialized genetic facilities are aware of patient's anxiety concerning the issue of confidentiality when it comes to their medical health records. Many patients fear that if the results of genetic testing become known, they may be fired from their jobs, face discrimination, or even be denied medical or life insurance policies. Be aware of the fact that the genetic tests and their results are considered confidential protected medical information, and your insurance company, your place of employment, and/or other individuals cannot have access to this information without your personal consent.

16. What is risk-reducing surgery?

After you have undergone genetic testing and reviewed the laboratory results with the genetic counselor and your medical doctor, you may decide that your risk for developing other cancers is much higher than the general population. Even though there are no signs of the particular type of cancer in your body, you may consider undergoing certain risk-reducing surgeries in order to help reduce your risks for future cancers. The two surgeries performed most often are risk-reducing bilateral salpingo-oophorectomy (removal of the ovaries and fallopian tubes) and a prophylactic mastectomy (removal of the breasts).

Bilateral salpingo-oophorectomy (RRBSO) is a surgical procedure that can often be done with a minimally invasive technique called **laparoscopy**, whereby the ovaries are surgically removed. This may be done on an outpatient basis or a short stay in the hospital. Removal of the ovaries can dramatically reduce your risks for ovarian cancer. Because the procedure is done laproscopically, with a tiny incision that heals fast, your hospital stay is minimal and you rarely miss a lot of time from work or other social obligations. After the ovaries are surgically removed, you will go into premature menopause (if you are not menopausal already) and most women will suffer from hot flashes and vaginal dryness. There may also be some impact on your bones. Some women relay a feeling of empowerment after performing this type of surgery because they are acting in a proactive fashion and confronting their risk of cancer head on. They are attempting to do everything within their power to stay as healthy as possible and prevent another type of cancer.

The **prophylactic mastectomy** is when the normal breast tissue is surgically removed in the unaffected breast to help minimize the risk of recurrence or the development of another new primary breast cancer. Very often, reconstructive or plastic surgeons can be on

Bilateral salpingo-oophorectomy (RRBSO)

the surgical term for removal of both the right and left fallopian tubes and ovaries.

Laparoscopy

camera-directed surgery done without creating a large incision into the abdomen.

Prophylactic mastectomy

when normal breast tissue is removed in the unaffected breast to help minimize the risk of recurrence or the development of another new primary breast cancer.

hand to perform immediate reconstruction of the breast. Implants can be placed or muscle and tissue flaps from other areas of the body can be used to reconstruct breasts. Nipples also can be reconstructed and sometimes tattooing can be used to create realistic appearing nipples on the breasts.

17. What are some of the signs of breast cancer? What can I do to reduce my risk for breast cancer?

Many women of all races, socioeconomic backgrounds, religions, and social standing will develop breast cancer over the course of their lifetime. According to the latest statistics from the National Cancer Institute, it is estimated that one in seven North American women will develop breast cancer in her lifetime. Breast health awareness is important so that you can maintain excellent breast health. Every woman should know the potentially troublesome indications that may signal breast disease.

There are a multitude of signs and symptoms that indicate breast cancer. Some of them include a single painless lump, swelling, or an unusual appearance of one or both breasts, thickening of the breast skin, a newly inverted nipple or bloody discharge from the nipple, a depression in the breast or a change in breast contour, nipple pain, scaliness, ulceration, or a sudden discharge from the nipple. A rash on the breast or nipple can also be suggestive of underlying malignancy. Every woman is at risk for developing breast cancer. It is important to know your personal family history. If breast cancer runs in your family, if you have had a previous abnormal breast biopsy, or if your male relative had breast cancer, you are at a greater risk for developing breast cancer. Other known risk factors include: long menstruation time (menstrual periods that started early in life and finish late), a genetic predisposition including the *BRCA1* and *BRCA2* genetic mutations (see Question 15), a breast biopsy that is confirmed for atypical hyperplasia, **obesity** after menopause, prolonged postmenopausal hormonal therapy (especially the use of estrogen and progesterone), never having had any children, first delivery after 30 years of age, and the consumption of more than one alcoholic beverage per day.

Obesity
the medical condition referring to a severely overweight patient.

Now that you are aware of some of the signs and risk factors for developing breast cancer, how can you modify your risk? While you certainly cannot change the fact that you are a woman, there are certain lifestyle changes that can possibly help reduce your risk for developing breast cancer.

Breastfeeding your child helps to reduce the risk for breast cancer and it provides important nutrients and immune-boosting proteins for your newborn. Several studies on breast cancer risk reduction clearly link the woman maintaining a correct body weight, reduced alcohol intake, and a vigorous exercise plan with a lowered risk for cancer development, particularly breast cancer. Limiting your alcohol intake to no more than one alcoholic beverage daily, maintaining your ideal body weight, and limiting saturated fats in your diet while exercising regularly helps with your general health maintenance and reduces your risk of cancer. An annual mammogram at a certified institution (one that is accredited to perform mammography) coupled with clinical breast exams by a physician and monthly

Breast self-examination (BSE)

the act of examining your own breasts on a monthly basis to detect any changes. BSE should be preformed in a variety of positions including standing, sitting, and lying down. Visual inspection of the breasts should also occur.

breast self-examinations (BSE) (see Question 19) are also key facets in maintaining breast health.

For some women who are at a high risk for the development of breast cancer, a drug called tamoxifen can be an option to help reduce breast cancer. Tamoxifen can reduce the risk of breast cancer recurrence, decrease its spread, and reduce the risk of cancer in the unaffected breast. Tamoxifen also may have an added benefit of helping to preserve bone health and lowering cholesterol levels; however, it can cause hot flashes, endometrial lining overgrowth (which can lead to uterine cancer), and research has shown that it may contribute to serious life-threatening blood clots. Every woman should balance the risks versus the benefits when deciding to take this medication and it is always important to consult with your breast healthcare provider before making any decisions.

Letrozole

an anti-estrogen type of medication.

Other medications called aromatase inhibitors like **Letrozole** (Femara®), Anastrazole (Arimidex®), and Exemestane (Aromasin®) are currently being used for the treatment of hormonally-sensitive breast cancer and may also be used as protective agents in the future. Recently, Novartis (manufacturer of Femara®) issued a label warning concerning this medication, stating that it should not be used as an ovulation agent because of the potential to cause fetal toxicity and malformations. It is important to mention that women who are on these adjunctive medications for breast cancer treatment may need contraception to prevent pregnancy. It is always best to consult your physician and discuss the issues with respect to the medication you may be prescribed.

Some of the myths concerning breast cancer should be dispelled. At the present time, there are no accurate scientific data that directly link underwire bras, antiperspirant usage (see Question 25), or having had an elective termination of pregnancy with breast cancer.

18. What should I know about breast cancer prevention?

Mammography (a special X-ray of the breast where the radiation exposure of the breast tissue is minimal), clinical breast examination by a physician, and breast self-examination are three of the best techniques to help detect breast disease at an early stage. All three contribute to excellent breast health. Even though eight out of ten breast lumps turn out to be non-cancerous, breast cancer detection and prevention are important parts of the general health maintenance program for the female cancer survivor.

It has been estimated that over 2 million breast cancer survivors are alive, well, and healthy in the United States today. The American Cancer Society recommends that women get annual mammograms beginning at the age of 40. After that mammograms should be repeated every one to two years until the age of 50, when they should to be done on an annual basis. The screening program should be individualized according to risk factors and family history. Breast self-examination for women over the age of 20 is also advocated on a monthly basis and clinical breast examination by a healthcare professional should be a part of the routine annual health maintenance examination.

Some women, especially those with a strong family history of breast cancer, may be candidates for earlier mammograms or breast ultrasound screening tests (see Question 15). Women with a strong family history of breast cancer or those with the *BRCA1* or *BRCA2* genetic mutations should begin surveillance at age 35 or up to 10 years before the diagnosis in the youngest affected relative. Some women who have had a history of radiation exposure to the chest as a result of whole body radiation may qualify for early mammogram screening as well. It is best to consult your physician and see if you are a candidate for an early mammogram or screening test. Some breast health authorities advocate that at-risk young women may be good candidates for magnetic resonance imaging and may recommend this test for these women.

Although during the mammogram the breast is compressed between two rigid plates and it may be uncomfortable, it is a relatively short test that is often completed in fifteen minutes. The mammogram can detect very small abnormalities in the breast even before they can be felt on a physical examination or by you during your breast self-examination.

On the day of your mammogram, it is important to remember that you should not use any deodorant or antiperspirant, as some contain certain ingredients that can interfere with correct interpretation of the mammogram. It is often more convenient to wear a two piece outfit, because you will need to be undressed from the waist up for the mammogram procedure. The best time to have a mammogram is shortly after your menstrual cycle. Always follow up and call your gynecologist or healthcare provider if you do not receive your mammogram results within a few days after the test. Some mammogram places will even give you the results immediately after the test is completed.

It may be helpful to ask for a copy of the mammogram report for your medical files or for your healthcare professional.

Other breast tests may be done for a variety of reasons. A breast ultrasound is an imaging technique that uses high-frequency sound waves to examine dense breast tissue; it is sensitive enough to distinguish between a cyst and a solid mass. Magnetic resonance imaging (MRI) uses strong magnets to enhance images to detect normal and abnormal blood flow patterns in different lesions in the breast and may be helpful in certain clinical situations. The MRI can construct a three-dimensional picture of the breast. Often, contrast dye is injected into your vein in order to improve image quality and picture development.

It is advisable to consult with your healthcare provider to determine what specific screening examination is necessary and which is best for you given your unique situation. No matter what screening technique you use, it is important to get annual mammograms and perform breast self-examination. Screening leads to early detection, which can save your life.

19. What is breast self-examination?

Women should be aware of how their breasts naturally appear and feel. Because early detection is the most crucial factor to surviving breast cancer, women who know their own bodies have a greater opportunity for discovering any changes. By the age of 20 or 21, a woman should be performing monthly breast self-examinations on a regular basis. Healthcare providers encourage women to examine their own breasts on a regular monthly basis, usually about three days after your menstrual cycle. If you are no longer having regular periods, choose an easy date to remember, such as your favorite number, your birthday date, or simply the first of every month, and examine your breasts on that specific day every month.

Some important aspects to remember for breast self examination (BSE)

- Examine your breast once a month in both the lying down and upright positions.
- Feel the entire breast for any lumps and check under your arm up to the level of your collar bone as well as below your breast.
- Examine the nipple and look for any changes in color or any fluid from the nipple. Any nipple scaliness or change in color should be reported. Gently squeeze the nipple; any discharge should also be documented and this should be reported to your breast clinician.
- You should always examine your breasts with your arms raised over your head and look for any changes in shape size or contour. Any puckering of the skin, changes in color or redness or abnormal discharge should be further evaluated. Then put your hands on your hips and examine the breasts again.
- Some women prefer examining their breasts before and after a shower. Others do it in front of a mirror or in the privacy of their bedroom.
- Use the middle pads of the middle three fingers and with light, medium, and hard pressure, check both breasts for any lumps or bumps.
- You can use either a circular pattern or rows, whatever you feel more comfortable doing. Make certain that you examine each entire breast. Some women use a light moisturizer or some body lotion on their

fingers during the examination. It may help them feel for any abnormalities better.

- If you feel something out of the ordinary, it is best to seek evaluation from a medical professional who may order further testing to assess the breast tissue.

(Adapted from Patient Educational materials from Memorial Sloan Kettering Cancer Center)

Most women find lumps themselves and the majority are not cancerous. Seeking help and evaluation in a timely fashion will often help get earlier treatment.

20. How can I prevent colon cancer? What is a colonoscopy?

According to the Cancer Research and Prevention Foundation, colon cancer is the second leading cause of cancer deaths in the United States. Close to 145,000 women and men are diagnosed and between 55,000 and 56,000 die each year from the disease. When discovered early, colon cancer is treatable and often curable.

According to the American Cancer Society, the accepted risk factors for developing colon cancer include: a personal or family history of colorectal cancer, colonic polyps, or having inflammatory bowel disease. Other risks may include alcohol consumption, smoking tobacco, inactivity, and consumption of large quantities of red meat because it is high in saturated fats. Women who take hormonal therapy or have a history of nonsteroidal anti-inflammatory drugs (NSAIDs; like aspirin) may be at a lower risk for developing colon cancer. Women on hormonal therapy also may be diagnosed at a later stage of the disease.

Colon cancer is a serious medical illness for women and most medical associations advocate colon screening starting at the age of 50. There are several methods to screen for colon cancer. Some include a *fecal occult blood test* where you will be given a home testing card kit. You are asked to get a sample of stool on the card, insert it into the supplied plastic sleeve and mail it to a laboratory. The card sample is then tested for the presence or absence of blood. Other tests are a flexible sigmoidoscopy (every 5 years), colonoscopy, and double-contrast barium enema. It is understandable that you may be fearful or embarrassed about the colon. But you must remember that rectal screening is one of the positive steps you can take toward disease discovery and early effective treatment.

Colonoscopy
a medical outpatient surgical procedure that is the screening tool to detect colonic abnormalities and precancerous growths in the colon.

A **colonoscopy** is a medical outpatient surgical procedure that is the screening tool to detect colonic abnormalities and precancerous growths in the colon. It looks at the large intestine or colon and rectum. It is the best type of test that can image the lining (colonic mucosa) and can be used to accurately identify colon cancer. After a special preparation that cleanses the colon, a small tube, which is thin and flexible and has a small video camera with a light source at the end, is placed within the rectum and advanced so that the gastrointestinal specialist can see the entire lining of the colon. The tube is lubricated so that it can be advanced into the colon with little discomfort. You will have received some sedation before the procedure, so you will be in a relaxed state of mind called "twilight." You will be conscious but unable to recall all of the details of the procedure.

Colonoscopies are typically done to investigate for bowel diseases, for example, changes in bowel function (diarrhea, constipation), bowel **polyps**, rectal bleeding, Chrone disease, and diverticulitis. Colonoscopies are an integral part of general health maintenance for adults over the age of 50 and should be part of a comprehensive screening protocol. Some women who are at particular risk for colon cancer, who may have a family history of hereditary non-polyposis colon cancer or other specific genetic predispositions, may be offered colonic screening at an earlier age.

Colonoscopy is a relatively safe and common procedure, but there are some minor risks associated with the procedure. You may have a reaction to the sedative that is given intravenously (injected into the bloodstream). There is also a small risk of infection, bowel perforation (a puncture in the intestinal wall that may require surgical intervention for repair), and bleeding. You may also experience some abdominal pain, discomfort, or fever following the procedure. Ask your doctor if you have some specific concerns or questions prior to beginning the procedure and before getting any sedating medications. If during the procedure the clinician sees a polyp or a suspicious lesion, the area can be biopsied (removed) for analysis and diagnosis. Colonic polyps can be removed during the colonoscopy. They appear in a variety of shapes and sizes; some are precursors to cancer but most often colonic polyps are benign (not cancer).

If you have any special medical concerns, like heart or lung diseases, artificial heart values, or have been instructed by other physicians or dentists to take antibiotics before surgical procedures, then you may be required to take antibiotics as well before your colonoscopy. If you are on *ANY* medications, it is best to discuss timing and dosages with your healthcare

Polyp

a projecting mass of swollen tissue that may appear in the intestine or on the cervix. Endometrial polyps occur within the uterine cavity. Most are benign.

General Health Maintenance

provider before your colonoscopy. Sometimes medications will be changed or not taken, while others can be taken as usual on the day of the procedure.

Before the day of the procedure, you will be asked to perform a bowel preparation. It may entail drinking large volumes of special fluids and not taking any food by mouth. This preparation is required to clean the colon so that the doctor may better visualize the cells lining the walls (mucosa). Once you arrive at the place where the procedure is to be done, you will be examined by a healthcare professional, who will ask details of your medical history and complete a physical examination. A **consent form** for the procedure will be reviewed with you before the procedure.

Consent form

a written document signed by a patient to indicate that someone (most likely their physician) has explained to the patient about a particular treatment, including its risks and benefits; signing the form means that the agrees to receive the treatment; also referred to as "informed consent."

During the colonoscopy, which can last from thirty minutes to one hour, you will be wearing a hospital gown and an intravenous drip containing some medications to make you sleepy or cause you to relax will be placed in your arm. You will feel sleepy and drowsy during the entire procedure. During the procedure, your vital signs (blood pressure, heart rate, and level of oxygen) will be monitored by special machines. Some people experience some side effects like mild cramping, bloating, or abdominal discomfort that usually subside with time.

After completing the procedure, you will be monitored in the recovery room or area and be expected to stay in there for some time before being allowed to go home. It is always advisable for you to have a family member or friend to help you travel home. You should expect to rest for the remainder of the day. Most physicians advocate no driving or using heavy machinery for several hours after the procedure, but it is always advisable to ask your gastrointestinal specialist for your specific discharge instructions and limitations. If you have had a biopsy or surgical removal of a polyp, ask your healthcare professional if there are any other specific, specialized post-biopsy instructions or certain activities you should limit. Also, ask if certain conditions should be looked out for, like rectal bleeding or spotting.

A virtual colonoscopy (sometimes called a computed tomography colography) is when you are screened for colon cancer by a noninvasive technique. You are placed in a computerized machine, either a magnetic resonance imaging (MRI) or computed tomorgraphy (CT), which will digitally examine the colon from outside the body and present a three dimensional image. No tube is placed completely within your rectum. However, the advance preparation for a conventional and virtual colonoscopy are the same. The images are examined for any pathology and, if there are polyps in your colon, the traditional type of colonoscopy must be preformed so that they can be removed.

21. What are the harmful effects from the sun?

The sun is very damaging to the skin. The American Cancer Society estimates that over one million cases of nonmelanoma skin cancers (defined below) occurred in 2005. But sun related effects are preventable if you take the appropriate precautions. While the sun provides some very important aspects, for example, it provides warmth, helps plants to maintain photosynthesis, and helps the human body to produce vitamin D, the negative ramifications from sun exposure are numerous. Sun tanning and burning while in the sun's rays can increase the risks for skin cancer, and many women still do not take the necessary precautions to protect themselves from sun damage.

People who are fair skinned or have a light complexion, those with a family history of skin cancer, and those with multiple moles or who have experienced severe sunburns as a child may be at an increased risk for skin cancers. Ultraviolet radiation from sun exposure also may contribute to eye damage and negatively influence the immune system. According to the National Safety Council, children tend to be at highest risk because sun burning during childhood can contribute to the increased risk of melanoma in later life.

Some of the problems from overexposure to the sun can be skin cancer, eye damage, skin wrinkling (photoaging), and immunosuppression.

Skin cancer

(a) *Basal cell carcinoma* usually appears on sun exposed surfaces like the face, ears, lips, and the nose. Basal cell carcinomas usually appear as a red patchy area but can be white, red, or pinkish in color. It may be crusty, like an open sore that will not heal, or it may be darker in color and have an irregular border. The lesions can be shiny or **translucent**, or may appear as a waxy area that bleeds easily with little trauma.

(b) *Squamous cell carcinoma*, the second most common type of skin cancer, tends to be more aggressive in that it can spread (metastasize) to other organs or

Translucent

a type of barrier that diffuses the passage of light.

parts of the body if untreated. This cancer is relatively slow growing, but if untreated may lead to death. Tumors appear on sun exposed parts of the body, including the face, neck, scalp, ears, shoulders, back, hands, and feet. It may be a rough, scaly patch of slightly raised skin that ranges in color from brown to red, and can grow up to an inch in diameter. Lips tend to be cracked, dry, scaly, and or pale or white in color. Often it appears as an open wound with an irregular edge that will not heal and sometimes bleeds.

(c) *Melanoma*, the most deadly and aggressive type of skin cancer, can spread rapidly to other parts of the body, and if untreated can be fatal. A normal mole is round and has the same color brown. One that is a melanoma is asymmetric (the two halves of the lesion are not the same), its borders are irregularly shaped, the color is different throughout the lesion, and the diameter is larger than 1/4 of an inch (6 mm; about the size of a pencil eraser). Over time it will evolve. This means that changes occur in color, size, shape, symptoms (itching, tenderness), and/or surface (excessive bleeding).

Eye damage

There is growing evidence that the sun's rays are harmful to the human eyes, which may contribute to the development of cataracts, a condition where the eye's lenses lose their transparency and develop a type of film that causes cloudy vision. According to the American Association of Ophthalmology, another potential effect of the sun is "burning" of the eye surface; often there is temporary pain that goes away when the person rests in a darkened room for several days. When this happens from the reflection of sunlight off of snow in high altitudes or near the polar circle, it is known as *snow blindness*. The sun's rays may also have a role in the development of *macular degeneration*, which is an incurable deterioration of the retina that leads to blindness (and occurs mostly in those aged over 55), and eyelid cancer.

Skin wrinkling or photoaging

Overexposure to the sun can lead to changes in the skin's elasticity and pliability, which may result in skin wrinkling. It contributes to a leathery texture of the skin surface. Other skin changes can include furrowing, liver spots, and bruising.

Immunosuppression

Exposure to the sun's rays and light can cause **immuno-suppression**, a condition that weakens the body's ability to fight disease. Some scientists believe that the sun may influence human white blood cell count.

Immuno-suppression

when the body's natural immune responses are lowered by drugs or an illness; this condition increases the body's susceptibility to infection.

22. What is sun health? What is dermatological screening?

Sun health involves actively protecting yourself from the sun's harmful rays and decreasing your risks from the adverse effects from the sun. Some helpful suggestions are listed below:

a) Limit sun exposure during the times when the sun is the most harmful, from 10 AM to 4 PM. It is always advisable to cover the sun exposed parts of your body with long sleeved, lightweight clothing. If possible, refer to the ultraviolet (UV) index in your area, which indicates the intensity of the sun's rays. Plan for indoor activities or avoid the outdoors when this index is unfavorable.

b) Shade! Shade! Shade! Seek shaded areas near trees or under the cover of an umbrella when you are outdoors. Wear hats with brims to help shield your face, ears, head and neck, and wear eye protection against the sun's damaging rays. Pick specially designed hats with a wide brim as they cast shadows and can offer additional coverage to other areas of the body. Carry an opened umbrella on a sunny day to help shield the sun from your face and body.

c) Keep your body's sensitive areas covered. Shirts and light colored pants are a must in hot sun because they can protect the skin from harmful rays. Remember to cover up when in the sun. The use of light fabrics that breathe (like cotton or rayon) can prevent overheating and limit the amount of perspiration. This way you can enjoy the outdoors and not expose yourself to harm.

d) Treat yourself to a pair of eyeglasses that can protect you from UV light. Check the UV index and be sure they are tested and approved for maximal sun protection. Eyeglasses that offer good sun protection also help protect the sensitive skin around your eyes and eyelids.

e) Avoid the sun altogether when it is a particularly hot and brightly sunny day. It is always helpful to plan indoor activities if possible to miss the midday oppressive heat.

f) Use sunscreen. The liberal use of a non-expired sunscreen that has a minimum sun protection factor (SPF) of 15 and can block both the UVA and UVB rays of the sun is essential. You should apply a sunscreen often and liberally, especially on sunny or cloudy/hazy days. Sunscreens should be applied approximately 30 minutes before exposure to the sun and should be applied repeatedly, especially when engaging in water sports, swimming, or other activities that cause a lot of perspiration. Most sunscreens have an expiration date so be careful when shopping for the best sunscreen and check the expiration date before purchasing these products. Throw away last year's products and purchase a new supply. Many companies now also have specialized lip balm with built-in sun protection and moisturizers that help protect your lips from the sun's damaging rays.

g) Tanning salons or parlors should be avoided because they can cause skin damage and lead to skin diseases. They may contribute to premature aging and wrinkling of the skin. A new psychiatric condition named Tanorexia occurs when either men or women are addicted to sun tanning; they obsess about either getting a tan in a salon or outdoors. This can be a serious and damaging medical condition where people can be obsessed and preoccupied with tanning despite the known detrimental effects that the sun can produce.

23. How should I care for my skin?

Estrogen receptors are found in various parts of the skin. When you have lowered estrogen levels because of menopause, treatment for cancer, or as a result of premature menopause, your skin may begin to show signs of thinning. Fibroblasts are specialized skin cells that have estrogen receptors but do not produce the same amount of protein or collagen as they used to. Skin may appear wrinkled, dry, and red or even have acne.

Some helpful suggestions for maintaining healthy skin during menopause include using a daily foaming cleanser that has a moisturizer, and for the shower use a moisturizing soap or body wash. Very hot water can affect the skin, so warm showers are best. Keeping your shower time to a minimum will prevent your skin from drying out. Moisturize your skin and use sun protection to prevent further damage. Many cosmetic products are specifically designed for the sensitive areas of the face. Diets filled with fruits and vegetables that are rich in antioxidants can also help skin integrity and elasticity. Smoke, tobacco, and second hand smoke all are very detrimental for your health and can age your skin prematurely. Lastly, water is important to keep your skin healthy and hydrated, so drink as much water as you can. It is recommended that you drink at least six to eight glasses of water per day.

A dermatological self-screening examination

A dermatological self-screening examination is when you examine your entire body from head to toe when naked, and note all moles lesions or discolorations on your body. An examination should be done frequently; some dermatologists advocate doing this twice a year.

Some women who have received high dosage radiation as part of their initial cancer therapy may be at an increased risk for developing malignant melanoma, so a skin evaluation is an important part of their annual physical examination. It is important to stand before a mirror and examine both the front and back portions of your body. Some people find it helpful to use a diary in which they can document the size, shapes, colors, and textures of their moles. Be certain to examine the back of your legs and scalp as well. Look in between toes and soles, and do not forget the neck region. Digital pictures can be taken and placed within the notebook for future reference.

Do this often so that you will become familiar with all the moles and small blemishes, spots, and dots on your body. If they change in shape, size, color, or begin to bleed, it is always best to seek a professional evaluation. If you are uncertain about a mole or are finding self-examination difficult, leave it to the professional dermatologist. Some dermatologists are now performing whole body digital photography to document moles and other bodily discolorations; in this way, they can monitor any changes to shape, size, color, or contour carefully as well as biopsy any suspicious lesions that have changed. For more information, contact the American Association of Dermatology (see Appendix), as they can be helpful in locating a skin screening facility with a reputable, board certified dermatologist who can assist you in maintaining good health skin care.

Apart from the health worries, what about the WRINKLES?! Come on, girls, slap on the sunscreen, wear your hat, and get your tan at the make-up counter. You don't want your face to look like a worn-out pocketbook, now do you?

Frances S.

BEHAVIOR AND SUBSTANCES

24. Should I avoid any substances or chemicals to lower my risk for cancer?

Several chemicals are well known to either cause or contribute to a person developing cancer. Some of the more well known substances include: **benzene,** a colorless liquid with a sweet odor that is formed from natural processes like forest fires. It is found in cigarette or cigar smoke, too. **Asbestos** is a fibrous material commonly used in insulation, floor tiles, textiles, and many other products until the mid-1980s. It has been associated with lung cancer and mesotheliomas (a type of cancer that affects cells lining organs that is a result of asbestos exposure). **Lead,** commonly found in household items such as paint and was a gasoline additive until the mid-1980s, when inhaled or ingested may cause many ill effects. Weakness, anemia, loss of appetite, vomiting, and convulsions are symptoms of lead toxicity that can lead to permanent brain injury and even death. **Tetrachlorethylene** is a chemical agent commercially produced for the dry cleaning industry and textile business; it is also used as a degreaser.

For more information concerning specific products and their potential for causing cancer, contact the American Cancer Society (see Appendix).

25. Do antiperspirants increase the risk for breast cancer?

According to the American Cancer Society, there is no good scientific evidence to support an association with **antiperspirant** use and the development of breast cancer. They cite a well designed study of over 800 breast

Benzene

a colorless, flammable liquid with a sweet odor formed from natural processes like forest fires; also found in cigarette and cigar smoke and is used in dry cleaning fabrics.

Asbestos

a fibrous silicate material formerly used in thermal insulation, floor tiles, textiles, and was valued for its strength and endurance in many other products. Studies have linked asbestos dust to the development of cancer.

Lead

commonly found in household items. When inhaled or ingested may cause many ill effects.

Tetrachlorethylene

a toxic agent commercially produced for the dry cleaning industry and textile business.

Antiperspirant

a cosmetic preparation used in the underarm area that controls excessive perspiration and odor.

cancer patients compared with healthy women that found no significant relationship or association of breast cancer and antiperspirant or deodorant use, or underarm shaving. Women are always advised not to wear antiperspirants on the day of their mammogram, because some of these products can contain aluminum that may appear as small flecks on the radiographic films. These specks can interfere with an accurate assessment of your mammogram.

26. Does talcum powder cause ovarian cancer?

Talcum powder is produced from talc, a mineral that in its natural form may contain asbestos. Since the 1970s, all talcum powders—including baby powder, facial, and body powders—were federally mandated to be asbestos-free. There is growing concern that talcum powder may be a carcinogen and thus associated with ovarian cancer. It is hypothesized that the talc travels from sanitary napkins, diaphragms, condoms, or genital sprays through the vagina, uterus, and fallopian tubes to adhere to the surface of the ovaries. Unfortunately, thus far scientific studies are confusing and mixed in their results. Some show an association of talc users with cancer when other studies fail to demonstrate an association. Because there is conflicting medical science regarding the linkage of talc and ovarian cancer, it seems prudent to avoid using substances that may contain talc and substitute powders for cornstarch-based material, which has not been shown in any studies to increase cancer risk.

27. Does my cellular phone cause brain cancer?

According to the Cellular Telecommunications and Internet Association, it is estimated that in 2004 there were over 170 million cellular phone users in the United States. Cellular telephones do not emit dangerous ionizing radiation; however, they operate using radio frequencies. The concern over brain cancer and the use of cell phones has gained popularity in the media recently. However, according to recent scientific studies, one done in Stockholm and the Uppsala region of Sweden, another conducted by the American Health Foundation, and a third completed by the U.S. National Institute, there was no definitive link between cell phone users and brain cancer. Patients with brain cancer did not report more cell phone use over control patients. No correlation between the side of phone use and the side of the brain cancer has been shown. There has been some interest in the possible association of cell phones and a rare brain tumor called acoustic neuromas. **Acoustic neuromas** are small, rare, slow-growing tumors that arise from the acoustic nerve, which is important for hearing. Currently, it is uncertain if the linkage of long-term cell phone use and acoustic neuromas is definitive.

In addition to concerns over cancer, cell phone use while driving an automobile has been definitively associated with an increased incidence of motor vehicle accidents. There is also growing concern that cellular phone use may interfere with medical electronic implantable devices such as **pacemakers** (which regulate the heart rate) or insulin pumps (which regulate blood sugar levels in diabetics). Because of the

General Health Maintenance

Acoustic neuromas

small, rare, slow-growing tumors that grow from the acoustic nerve (the nerve that is important for hearing).

Pacemaker

an electrical device that is surgically implanted into the chest that is used for stimulating or steadying the heart beat.

conflicting data about the absolute safety of cell phones, it seems prudent to advise people to limit the number of hours spent on the phone. The use of a wireless headset device with increased distance between the base of the phone and your body also seems like a practical solution to minimize your exposure to radio frequency energy. Updated cellular telephone information is available from two agencies:

Federal Communications Commission
RF Safety Program. Office of Engineering and Technology
http://www.fcc.gov/oet/rfsafety

Food and Drug Administration
Cell Phone Facts: Consumer Information on Wireless Phones
http://www/fda.gov/cellphones/

28. What is diethylstilbestrol? Does it cause pelvic or genital cancer?

Diethylstilbestrol (DES) is a synthetic estrogen compound that was prescribed to women who had previous miscarriages or premature deliveries from the 1930s to the early 1970s. Its use fell out of favor in the 1960s when its efficacy came into question. Some scientific studies linked it to harmful effects on the reproductive tract of the developing fetus. Both women who took the medication and her offspring are at an increased risk for different types of pelvic cancers, and they should be followed in comprehensive cancer centers.

Women who took this medication may be at an increased risk for developing breast cancer. These women may benefit from close breast surveillance programs, digital mammograms, and clinical and breast self-examinations. Daughters of women who took DES are also at an increased risk for developing other cancers, including clear cell adenocarcinoma of the cervix or vagina. This is an extremely rare type of genital cancer. Daughters of women who took this medication should make certain to get an annual examination by a gynecologist or a **gynecological oncologist**. The National Cancer Institute has published guidelines that recommend yearly Pap smear tests and a pelvic examination as well as visual inspection that will look for abnormal cells. Women who were exposed to DES in utero also may experience other serious medical complications. These may include: structural changes in the vagina, cervix and uterus; fertility problems as well as an increased premature birth rate; increased ectopic or **tubal pregnancy** rate; and an increased incidence of spontaneous miscarriage. If you took this medication or you are a child of someone who supposedly took this medication while they were pregnant with you, it is best to consult your gynecological healthcare professional to discover if you are at increased risk for medical problems. Your gynecological specialist can facilitate getting you into a proper surveillance program and will make certain that you get the correct screening tests that will detect disease early if it may appear. For those who wish to obtain more information, contact DES Action USA (http://www.desaction.org, 1-800-DES-9288) or the DES Cancer Network, (http://www.descancer.org).

Gynecological oncologist

a degreed, certified physician specializing in the treatment of cancer of the female reproductive system.

Tubal pregnancy

a type of pregnancy where the egg has implanted in the fallopian tube instead of the uterus. This can be a serious medical condition and needs immediate medical attention.

29. Does cooking on my backyard barbeque cause cancer?

Health hazards from your summer backyard barbeque are well known and grilling food can now be considered a risk for your developing cancer. However, this risk does change depending on what and how you grill. With conventional food grilling of red meat, chicken, or seafood, a reaction between the food's protein and the high heat occurs that form carcinogenic compounds called *heterocyclic amines* (HCAs). These HCAs can damage the building blocks of our genes (the deoxyribonucleic acid) and start the process that can lead to the development of cancer, most commonly cancer of the stomach or colon.

One recent scientific study found that men and women who eat the most barbecued red meat (beef, pork, and lamb) almost doubled their risk of colon polyps compared to those who did not eat these foods grilled. There is also emerging evidence that the HCA can enter the bloodstream and affect other tissues, thereby possibly causing other types of cancer.

According to the American Institute for Cancer Research in Washington, D.C., some practical suggestions to avoid or minimize the risks of HCA is by grilling at lowered temperatures, thus decreasing the amount of HCAs that are created in your food. Try roasting your meats, and turn down the gas flame on your barbeque. Wait until the charcoal has become low-burning embers or turn down the level of the gas before you place your food on the grill to be cooked. Also, raise the grilling surface from the heat source. By doing so, you will lessen the amount of black char on the food, which has a high carcinogenic content.

Some other suggestions to reduce the amount of HCA content for your food include flipping your meat every minute and using a marinade. Marinating can decrease HCA formation by up to 96%. Another type of carcinogenic compound is called *polycyclic aromatic hydro-carbons* (PAHs). PAHs form when smoke is deposited on the outside of meat. By choosing leaner cuts of meat that have less fats, there will be less drip and fewer smoky flares. Be careful of always eating meat or poultry that is well done, because this type of meat consumption has been linked with two to five times more colon cancer and two to three times more breast cancer. The risk for developing cancers of the stomach and pancreas may also increase.

Most healthy nutritional diet plans (see Questions 32–36) suggest limiting the amount of red meat, and the American Institute for Cancer Research recommends limiting consumption of all red meat to no more than three ounces a day. You can limit your risk by choosing marinated lean chicken breasts or fish to grill for your summer barbeque party. You can always choose a healthy selection of vegetables to grill as well; try some veggie kabobs. Vegetables don't form HCAs and these foods also supply a whole range of cancer-fighting nutrients and antioxidants.

30. I know that smoking tobacco causes cancer. How can I get help to stop smoking?

Health problems associated with smoking are well known. There is a strong association of a variety of cancers with tobacco use. Lung, throat, and tongue cancers are all associated with tobacco smoking. Smoke has also been associated with kidney, bladder, voice box (larynx), and cervical cancer, and even some types of leukemia. Cigarette smoking does contribute to a variety of medical illnesses, including emphysema, bronchitis, peripheral vascular disease, and cardiac illness.

The components of smoke—nicotine and tar—affect blood vessels by promoting plaque build up in arteries, which contributes to cardiovascular disease. Smoking is also a risk factor for cervical cancer. Inhaling second hand smoke is also harmful to your health and should be avoided. You should encourage others who smoke not to do so in your presence, and make your home and office a smoke-free zone.

Most cancer institutions, including the American Cancer Association, have formalized smoking cessation programs that can help you stop smoking if you have not done so already. Some of the nicotine replacement options are a patch, inhaler, chewing gum, or spray. The side effects of nicotine replacement therapy include: headaches, dizziness, stomach upset, visual changes, unusual dreams or nightmares, or diarrhea. The medication bupropion (Zyban®) also can be used to help someone quit smoking. Although it is classified as an **antidepressant** medication, it can be used in combination with nicotine replacement therapy and a formalized smoking cessation program.

Antidepressant
a type of medication used to decrease the symptoms of low mood (depression).

Many smoking cessation programs tailor the curriculum to the specific individual and often offer a combined approach of medications, nicotine replacement therapy, hypnosis, and counseling. The combined treatment of smoking with many modalities helps smokers stop this unhealthy habit permanently.

It is clear that smoking poses serious medical problems, including its contribution to cancer and cardiovascular disease. Make a date to quit today and begin living an active and healthy life!

I think that quitting smoking is harder than all the Sunday New York Times *crossword puzzles put together. Harder than calculus. Don't give up. Just keep trying until you quit for good. And when you are ready, you will. You will. And it's only really hard for a short time, I promise.*

Frances S.

31. What should I know about my alcohol consumption?

Although moderate amounts of alcohol consumption have been linked to a decrease in cardiovascular disease, drinking more than two alcoholic beverages per day is associated with increased risks for developing breast cancer and other diseases. According to the American Cancer Society, excessive alcohol consumption has been linked to a variety of cancers including cancer of the tongue, esophagus, pharynx, larynx, and liver. It is estimated that women who drink two to five alcoholic beverages daily have a one and a half times higher risk of developing breast malignancy. Alcohol also contributes to poor bone health or osteoporosis, and may raise blood pressure.

It is easy to become confused about this issue because you probably have heard reports that a single alcoholic beverage is beneficial for cardiovascular health for men over age 50 and women over 60. It is always best to consult your healthcare provider to weigh the balance between cardiovascular benefit and risk for cancer when it comes to alcohol consumption.

Important facts to remember are that one alcoholic beverage is defined as a regular 12-ounce beer, a

5-ounce glass of white or red wine, or 1.5 ounces of 80 (percent) proof hard liquor (such as scotch, bourbon, gin, vodka, etc.). Pregnant women, young children, and young teens who have not reached the drinking age should never consume alcohol. It is also important to know that alcohol does interfere with many prescription medications and does impact your ability to react quickly as it slows down your reflexes. Last but not least, if you have had something alcoholic to drink, it is always best to avoid driving an automobile or operating dangerous equipment. Moderation is the rule with alcohol consumption.

PART 3

Nutrition

What are some healthy foods to include in my diet?

Will taking vitamins help my health?

How can I use complementary therapies, such as herbs, to help my general health?

More . . .

Interest in food, including smells, taste, and thinking about eating an enjoyable meal are often the first signs that you are entering the survivorship phase of your healing process. Cancer patients often suffer from nausea, dry mouth, metallic tastes, vomiting, and loss of appetite during the therapy for their cancer. Now that you are a survivor, foods will begin to be more appealing. You may be seeking out foods that you previously had avoided. Eating well will help you regain your strength, stamina, and augment your overall health. Do discuss any food restrictions with your healthcare professional.

Goals of good nutrition
- To optimize your general well being and health
- To improved your quality of life
- To achieve and maintain your correct body weight
- To boost and fortify your immune system

A proper diet rich in fruits, vegetables, and fortified grains helps you to combat fatigue and boosts your energy levels. As most North Americans tend to overeat, it is also important to learn what exactly is a correct portion, that is, what and how much is sufficient to eat. The content of food fat within some of your favorite foods is also important information to know. You can consult a local nutritionist or dietician to help you construct a healthy diet filled with cancer-reducing foods. A food specialist can also help you calculate portion size and the exact number of calories that are required for your unique and specific diet. A healthy diet includes all the basic food groups, which contain a balance of protein, carbohydrates, fats, minerals, and vitamins.

Protein is helpful for your immune function as it helps to repair body tissues. Some examples of protein are lean meats, fish, poultry, nuts, dried beans, and foods that contain soy. *Carbohydrates* digest quickly, supplying the body with a large portion of your energy requirements to function on a daily basis. Fruits, vegetables, pastas, grains, and cereals are all sources of carbohydrates.

According to the *2005 ACS Facts and Figures* booklet, the American Cancer Society recommends the following tips about nutrition and exercise for those who want to reduce their risk of developing cancer.

1) Eat a variety of healthy foods with an emphasis on plant sources.

   a) Eat five or more servings of fruits or vegetables daily.

   b) Choose whole grains instead of processed or refined grains and sugars.

   c) Limit consumption of high saturated red meats.

   d) Choose foods that help maintain a healthy weight.

2) Adopt a physically active lifestyle (see Questions 37–41).

   a) Adults should engage in 30 minutes of moderate exercise on at least five or more days of the week. Forty-five minutes of vigorous activity on five or more days further reduces colon and breast cancer risks.

   b) Children and adolescents should engage in 60 minutes of moderate to vigorous activity daily.

3) Maintain a healthy body weight throughout life.

a) Focus on weight reduction if overweight or obese.

b) Balance intake of foods with physical activity and exercise.

4) If you do drink alcoholic beverages, limit your consumption (see Question 31). Moderation is the rule.

a) Women should limit their consumption to no more than one alcoholic beverage per day.

32. What healthy foods should I include in my diet?

Beans.   No matter what the type of bean (legume) you eat, beans are an excellent source of dietary fiber, folate, magnesium, and vitamin B. They can help with constipation and may help lower your risk of cardiovascular disease. Some tasty beans include garbanzo, pinto, navy, kidney, and lentils. Other nutrients found in beans can help maintain a healthy lifestyle and reduce the risk of cardiovascular disease, diabetes, cancer, and osteoporosis. Diets high in fiber also can decrease cholesterol levels, heart disease, and blood pressure.

Berries.   Strawberries, blueberries, blackberries, and raspberries are excellent fruits to include in a healthy daily diet. They are a delicious treat and low in calories. They are an excellent source of antioxidants. Some scientific studies done in people who consume a lot of berries show that they have improved memory function and so scientists believe that eating berries may counteract aging memory loss. Cranberry and blueberry juices help to prevent urinary tract infections because bacteria cannot stick to the walls of the bladder and multiply to cause an infection. Cranberry juice may also act as a natural antibiotic to the urinary tract system.

Fruits. Most fruits contain vitamin C, antioxidants, folic acid, and are high in fiber, which helps you to maintain a healthy immune system. They add carbohydrates, which are nature's energy source. It is also important to include ripe fruits in a well balanced diet. Some that are important include the kiwi, which is an excellent source of vitamin C. Bananas are a good source of potassium. Five to seven servings of fruits and vegetables per day are recommended by the American Cancer Society's nutritional guidelines for cancer prevention.

One serving of fruit would include a medium sized apple or orange (the size of a tennis ball), one cup of raw vegetables cut up, a small handful of dried fruit, or five to six baby carrots. Fruits like cantaloupe, and some dark orange vegetables like sweet potatoes, carrots, and winter squash as well as red peppers contain vitamin A, which is known for its antioxidant (anti-aging) effects. Vitamin A is important for good vision and boosting the immune system function. Dried fruit is an excellent and easy snack food that you can take with you to the office. Pack a small plastic bag of fresh cut veggies such as celery or carrots and keep them in your desk as a midafternoon snack food! Always remember to wash your fruits and vegetables well before eating them.

Cereals. Cereals help to combat heart disease. They are high in fiber, which helps sweep waste out of your colon, softens your stool, and helps you prevent constipation. This action also helps you to maintain a healthy weight. Cereals help to lower cholesterol levels as well. Bypass media hype and read the nutrition labels on the packages. Avoid highly sugared and processed cereals; the ones you choose should not contain saturated fats, dyes or artificial flavors, or chemical preservatives. Choose whole grain (not "multigrain") cereals that are labeled "whole wheat" or "wheat bran" instead of just "wheat." (Also include whole grain breads in your diet.) Try combining cereals with yogurt instead of milk for added protein. Cooked whole grain cereals such as oatmeal (not cracked) are great tasting and nutritious. You can also sprinkle other types of whole grains on your regular cereal. Try bran buds! A sprinkle of amaranth adds protein and lysine; quinoa adds iron; barley adds fiber; millet adds folic acid; and whole grain rye adds vitamin E. A pinch of flaxseed, which has a nutty flavor, in addition to adding fiber, includes very important omega-3 essential fatty acids (EFAs). EFAs are building blocks for cell walls, cell signaling, and our neurological (brain and nerves) system, and studies show that they have a key role in helping to prevent many chronic diseases such as cardiovascular and neurological diseases.

Eggs. At a mere 68 calories, a single egg is a low cost source of high-quality protein. It contains choline and vitamin B_{12}, important nutrients for health. At one time, scientists recommended that we limit eggs in our diets because of the high cholesterol in the egg yolk. More exacting studies now show that it is the cooking oil (saturated fats) that produces higher cholesterol than two eggs. Those on a low fat diet can have one or two eggs per day without the risk of higher levels of cholesterol.

Leafy Green Vegetables. These are high in folate, a nutrient necessary for new cell growth. Leafy greens can help aid metabolism, maintain healthy bowel function, and enrich your diet of much needed nutrients like vitamin K, vitamin C, and folate. Cabbage may contain some anticancer properties known as glucosinolates. In a recent Polish women's health study, women who consumed about 30 pounds of cabbage a year were found to have a 72% lowered cancer risk. Broccoli is another delicious vegetable that is high in calcium and may boost cancer fighting enzymes. Collard greens, broccoli, cabbage, leafy green lettuce, and spinach should be included in every woman's diet. Vegetables with bright colors like yellow, red, or green have an abundant amount of nutrients and should be included in your diet.

Milk. An excellent source of calcium, milk may help with bone health and prevent bone loss; it also may promote healthy teeth. Other sources of high calcium include cheese, yogurt, salmon, broccoli, and fortified orange juice. Try 1% or skim milk rather than whole milk to reduce your fat intake. Calcium is an important nutrient for a woman throughout her life.

Nuts. Nuts are high in vitamin E, which may lower cholesterol levels. They are full of omega-3 fatty acids, folic acid, copper, arginine, calcium, and fiber. Walnuts, cashews, hazelnuts, macadamias, pecan, pistachio, pumpkin seeds, almonds, or pine nuts are excellent choices. Include them as snack foods. They can be easily made into small packages for your purse, lunch bag, or briefcase. Be careful if you buy prepackaged assorted nuts because some are liberally coated with salt, which can increase your blood pressure.

Fish and Meat. Cold oily fish contain omega-3 fatty acids, which combats cardiovascular and many other diseases (EFAs are discussed above). Salmon is not the only fish in the cold oily family. Anchovies, bluefish, herring, flounder, and mackerel are tasty choices. Consult your local fish market or the Food and Drug Administrations about any health advisories in your area about the mercury content and safety of certain types of fish. Replacing red meats that are high in fat or those that are cured or processed (beef, bacon, sausages, salami, bologna, etc.) with lowered fat and healthy fish selections makes healthy dietary sense. Choose lean cuts of meat that have a low fat content. Always trim off excess visible fat. Avoid fatty cuts of beef or pork, and choose poultry or fish instead.

Water. Most people do not drink enough fluids throughout the day, but water is vital for our good health. Our bodies are about 60% to 70% water. Blood is mostly water and our brains, lungs, and muscles all need plenty of water to function. Water regulates our internal temperature, carries oxygen and nutrients to the cells, and flushes out waste products. We lose water through sweat, urination, and our breath (respiration). Chronic joint and muscle pain, lower back pain, headaches, and constipation are all symptoms of mild dehydration. You need water long before you are thirsty.

The best source is regular drinking water. Sodas contain unnecessary sugar, artificial coloring, sweetening agents, and other chemicals. Other beverages like those that contain caffeine (such as coffee and tea) and alcohol do not count towards your daily intake. Sports drinks that contain electrolytes also are high in calories and sugar. If you can not stand the taste of plain water or find it bland and unappealing, add a lemon or lime wedge to get a zesty flavor.

33. Is it okay to use herbs?

Yes, many herbs have centuries of history of adding flavors to foods as well as wonderful health benefits. Traditional Chinese, Tibetan, and the Ayurevedic (India) systems of medicine have ancient histories and are used worldwide. An herb is typically all or a part of a particular plant that has been ground into a powder or boiled as a decoction. In the United States, herbal supplements are not FDA (Federal Drug Administration) regulated and most have not been extensively scientifically studied.

It is important to note that some herbs may interfere with prescription or over-the-counter medications. Talk with your medical or surgical oncologist and research in your local library and/or on the Internet before taking any herbal remedy. Memorial Sloan Kettering Cancer Center's Web site (http://www.mskcc.org/aboutherbs/) and the National Institute of Health's National Center for Complementary and Alternative Medicine (http://www.nccam.nih.gov) are excellent sources of objective, current information concerning the benefits and side effects of herbs.

Several herbs are now under intense scientific study. Ginkgo biloba may reduce the risk for developing ovarian cancer, according to a recent study conducted at Michigan State University. Garlic is widely known to help decrease the risk of developing cancer and it has added benefits of lowering blood pressure and cholesterol levels. For centuries, garlic has been used as an antibacterial agent. Turmeric, a yellow mustard spice, has been the subject of a scientific study by M.D. Anderson Cancer Center (Houston, Texas). Curcumin, a compound derived from turmeric, may enhance the effectiveness of some chemotherapy drugs and decrease the likelihood of breast cancer metastasis.

Green Tea.   In the Far East, green tea has long been known for its medicinal properties to energize and boost the immune system. Green tea contains powerful antioxidants. The National Cancer Institute has funded a clinical trial in humans at the Mayo Clinic (Rochester, Minnesota) to determine if a green tea extract can kill leukemia cells. These same researchers already published research data concerning the green tea extract, *epigallocatechin gallate*, which in the laboratory decreased the proteins that prolong the chronic lymphoblastic leukemia cells.

Beware of packaging labeled "natural" and "healthy." Educate yourself about reading labels and about nutrition in general. Two of the best books out there are Eat to Live, *by Joel Fuhrman and Mehmet Oz, and* Ultra Prevention, *by two highly respected Canyon Ranch physicians, Mark Hyman and Mark Liponis.* Ultra Prevention, *by the way, is about nutrition and a host of other health issues, written in an upbeat, positive (but not to say Pollyanna) tone. About five people gave it to me after the diagnosis. It's full of good information. It's empowering. It's hopeful.*

Frances S.

34. Should I take vitamin supplements or mega doses of vitamins to help my health?

According to a recent article in *The Wall Street Journal*, it is estimated that up to 70% of North Americans purchase vitamin supplements, spending a surprising $7 billion per year. However, as with many herbs (see Question 33), there are few well-controlled scientific studies showing a proven benefit. In fact, when taken in high doses, many vitamins can cause physical illness or interfere with medications you are taking. Taking an excess of vitamins (so-called "mega" vitamin dosages) may be dangerous to your health and also may cause serious side effects.

One vitamin myth is about beta carotene, which was promoted as a cancer-fighting agent. Later studies showed that it may contribute to lung cancer in some smokers. Vitamin A is thought to be an important factor in vision and immune system. But according to a 2002 Harvard University study of over 70,000 nurses who took high levels of vitamin A either in their regular diet or in supplement form, excess hip fractures were found. Also, pregnant women should never consume excess doses of vitamin A because it has been associated with birth defects.

Vitamin E was thought to be beneficial for coronary disease, prostate health, and Alzheimer disease. Recent reports found that excess vitamin E may be associated with higher rates of congestive heart failure. The *University-Berkley Wellness Letter* no longer advocates vitamin E supplementation. A clinical trial from John Hopkins University demonstrated that people taking higher doses of vitamin E (greater than 400 IU) increased their risk of death by 4%. Although this study is controversial, a more recent study has linked vitamin E consumption to an increased risk of heart failure. Vitamin E may also negatively influence the effectiveness of conventional cancer therapies according to a study in head and neck cancer patients. An increased risk of recurrence of their cancer was found in those who took vitamin E instead of a placebo (a pill with no active medication or ingredient in it).

Vitamin C has been widely used to combat or prevent the common cold and many Americans consume excessive amounts of this vitamin in the hopes of maintaining good health. Unfortunately, the scientific data do not support its use except for shortening the duration of cold symptoms. A 2001 research study showed that cancer cells may develop resistance to conventional chemotherapy after being exposed to certain vitamins. In 2005, an article published in *Cancer Journal* stated that cancer patients should avoid antioxidant supplementation (including vitamin C) because cancer cells have been known to eat vitamin C and grow. The *Wall Street Journal* cited Dr. D'Andrea, a highly respected medical oncologist from Memorial Sloan-Kettering Cancer Center, as stating, "It's a mistake to think that cancer cells don't like nutrients." Although we are not completely certain medically that excessive vitamins nourish and promote cancer cells to grow, it seams prudent to enjoy a healthy, well balanced diet to get all your daily vitamin requirements.

The Women's Health Initiative cited that calcium with vitamin D may be beneficial in the prevention of bone fractures; however, this study noted an increased incidence of kidney stones. North American women tend not to take enough calcium in their diets because they tend to shy away from foods they believe are fattening, such as yogurt, cheese, and milk products. Calcium supplementation may be helpful for this patient population. It is true that the efficiency of calcium supplementation has come under fire recently; many studies failed to show any improvement in bone or general health. However, well balanced diets with foods rich in a variety of nutrients, food groups, vitamins, and minerals are the nutritional goal!

Because the data about vitamin use and mega supplements are controversial and conflicting, and some of the vitamins that have been advocated as antioxidants may in fact counteract or negatively affect conventional cancer therapies or even encourage cancer cell growth, it seems wise to be cautious concerning additional vitamin use or supplementation.

As stated in Question 34, it is always best to discuss your intentions to add vitamins with your healthcare team and nutritionist. By modifying your diet to increase the variety of fresh foods you eat, you can get all of your daily nutritional requirements.

35. What foods should I avoid to maximize my health benefits from my diet?

Weight is often measured by calculating your body mass index (BMI), and keeping an optimum goal of a BMI less than 25 (see Question 8). If your BMI is over 25, you may wish to consider making a few lifestyle changes to modify your daily habits. The following suggestions can help you to lose weight or may help you improve your already healthy nutritional plan (see Questions 37–41 for tips about exercising).

1. Broil or bake. Don't deep fry.
2. Avoid adding extra salt to your food.
3. Limit the amount of oil, butter, heavy cream, and fatty mayonnaise that you add to your food during preparation or cooking. Limit the amount on sandwiches.
4. Limit the consumption of deep fried potatoes (chips and fries) and other snack foods that are high in saturated fats and empty calories.
5. Sweets such as pies, cakes, cookies, and deep fried donuts can be very fattening. Although very tasty, pastries are filled with saturated fats.

6. Avoid eating blackened meats, including charcoal grilled or burnt foods.

7. Avoid cured meats or pickled food. Limit the amount of bacon, sausage, hot dogs, pepperoni, bologna, and other fatty cuts of ground beef. Trim off all of the excess fat you can see before cooking.

8. Limit alcohol consumption and avoid excessive intake altogether.

9. Eat less! Watch your portion size. Consciously cut down on the amount you are eating at a single sitting. When eating out at restaurants, cut back on the amount you order or immediately split the meal into a take home box for the next day. Skip or share the appetizer. Limit or eliminate the dessert. Eat slowly, chew thoroughly, and stop before you feel full. Never overeat!

10. Exercise more. Find creative ways to add steps into your regular routine. Take the stairs instead of the elevator; park your car further away from your office, grocery store, or shopping mall. Rake the leaves, garden, go on long walks, bike, and play outdoors with the entire family instead of watching television or sitting in front of a computer screen (see Questions 37–41).

11. Write down obtainable practical goals. Realize that weight control is a life-long commitment. It requires that you examine your physical and emotional relationships with food. Changing your eating habits may be difficult at first but the rewards are improved health, a firmer physique, and a boost in vitality.

12. Be realistic in your goals of food and weight loss. If you are obese or severely overweight, do not be

embarrassed to discuss your concerns with your doctor. Many new and safe prescription medications are available that may be helpful. For a small set of people who are severely obese, there is even surgery.

Other helpful suggestions from the Mayo Clinic include:

1. When preparing and serving meals, don't place serving bowls on the table. Food on the table encourages second helpings and grazing on what's left in the bowl. Place a small but reasonable portion on your plate and leave the rest of the food in the kitchen. That will limit returning for second helpings.

2. Slow down during mealtime. Take your time eating and chew every bite. Eating quickly fools the brain into thinking you are still hungry. By letting your brain catch up to your stomach, you will eat slower and less quantity in the long run.

3. Avoid outside distractions like television, reading, or working during mealtime. This helps you to focus only on eating rather than your attention being on something else, and before you know it you will have eaten more than you desired. Mealtime can be a time for the family to catch up on daily events and a special time for sharing.

4. Eat your salad and vegetables before the main course. These are low in calories and high in nutrients. They will fill you up so you won't splurge unnecessarily on your main course.

5. Drink plenty of water between bites. Remember to stop when you feel full. Stop even if there is food left on your plate!

Specialized diets

If you look at *The New York Times'* best sellers list, there will always be a book title with the latest trend in diet and exercise. A few of the more recent popular diet titles include: *Sugar Busters*, *Fit For Life*, *Atkins Diet Revolution*, the *South Beach Diet*, and *The Zone*. There are even soup and watermelon diets. Many diets are very strict and difficult to follow. Some do not have any medical foundation. Others vary food groups with some avoiding carbohydrates and others advocating a complete protein diet with little or no carbohydrates. Some propose eating a low calorie and high protein plan and others allow enormous amounts of fats. The Sugar Busters diet has you avoid insulin-creating types of foods like carrots and potatoes.

All diets have some things in common. They couple a decreased caloric intake with increased exercise so when the amount of calories entering the body is less than your expenditure, you will lose weight. No matter what diet you choose, it is important to consult with your physician or nutritionist as many are not actually nutritious and can be very hard to follow on a long-term basis. Often your initial loss of weight is actually a decrease in your body water content. This means that when you go off of the diet's strict regimen, not only will you gain your original weight back but you may pack on even more pounds later!

An excellent nutritional plan will fit into your schedule, supply you with a variety of foods in small portions, be balanced for all of your body's needs (vitamins, minerals, fiber) as well as satisfy your taste buds. The idea is to eat for life.

36. How can complementary therapies, nutriceuticals, vitamins, or supplements help my general health?

Many women choose complementary remedies, herbs, and vitamins to help maintain or improve their physical, mental, and general well being. It is best to discuss any of these choices with your physician before starting on it. Many supplements or herbs can have adverse health effects and some may interfere with chemotherapy (see Questions 32, 33, and 34). Others may interact with prescription medications. Memorial Sloan Kettering Cancer Center has an excellent integrative medicine division and has a useful Web site that provides abundant information concerning herbs and various supplements. It is also important to note that many herbs and vitamins have not yet been formally studied in well designed randomized control trials. Their efficacy in cancer survivors lacks specific medical and scientific proof. Unfortunately, a comprehensive review of all herbs and supplements is beyond the scope of this section. Because many can have serious toxic effects, it's always advisable to consult with your healthcare provider before starting any herbs or supplements.

Echinacea (*Echinacea purpura, Echinacea angustifolia,* and *Echinacea pallia*), available in tea or capsules, is an herb thought to reduce the symptoms of a common cold. It should not be used if you are allergic to ragweed, daisies, sunflowers, or are taking an immunosuppressive medication. Zinc lozenges have been heralded to reduce the duration and severity of the common cold but they can be toxic if taken in excess. St John's wort, a common herb often used for its antidepressant characteristics, may interfere with chemotherapy. Ginger helps relieve nausea; however, it does have some blood thinning properties, so if you are already on blood thinner medications or have been told by your healthcare providers to avoid aspirin and aspirin-like products, it is best to avoid ginger. Garlic may also lower fat, cholesterol levels, and blood pressure but it can also act as an anticoagulant and thus increase your risk for bleeding.

PART 4

Exercise

Why should I exercise?

How do I develop an exercise plan that works for me?

How can I overcome my resistance to
a more active lifestyle?

More ...

37. Why should I exercise?

According to *Pause* magazine (winter 2005 issue), exercise is an integral part of a general health maintenance plan. Exercise has been linked to decreased hot flashes, improved cardiac function, weight and stress reduction, and it may help lower your risk for certain cancers including breast cancer. Exercise may also help in your general feelings of well being. It can decrease your risk of stroke, colon cancer, and diabetes, and it can help lower your blood pressure. A balanced exercise plan can help keep your body, mind, and spirit healthy. Depression, lowered mood, and feelings of anxiety can be lessened with persistent exercise.

Flexibility, joint mobility, and weight bearing exercises should be a part of every woman's exercise regime. A good plan can help maintain bone health and may lessen the effects of osteoporosis. Exercise can improve body fitness and can minimize some adverse effects of cancer therapy such as nausea, fatigue, and sleep disturbances. Despite the numerous benefits of exercise, too many women fail to find the needed time for this healthy activity.

According to the American Cancer Society, several medical studies support the notion that exercise is actually healthy for recovering cancer patients. One study reported that those cancer patients who exercised reported having less fatigue than those who remained sedentary (not active). This same article included other health benefits of exercise: decreased depression, increased self-confidence, and higher levels of physical independence. Another study in the *Journal of Strength and Conditioning* stated that exercise for cancer survivors increased their strength, endurance, flexibility, and ultimately their relaxation. Still another recent study showed that women with breast cancer who participated in a vigorous exercise regime had a lowered incidence of cancer recurrence. Clearly, the medical and scientific literature strongly supports exercise as being safe and beneficial to your health.

A well balanced exercise plan can enhance your self-esteem while helping you maintain a normal body weight. Your blood circulation improves, endurance strengthens, blood pressure lowers, excess fatty deposits disappear, it helps with your balance, and improves joint stability and strength. After a regimen of exercise, you may rest better, have lower stress levels, and have much more energy to enjoy life's activities. It is never too late to start! Consult your doctor today and begin your healthy journey with some exercise (see Question 38).

38. What is an exercise plan? How do I get started?

According to the United States *2005 Dietary Guidelines for Americans*, a healthy exercise program should include cardiovascular exercises, weight training, and activities that involve stretching, flexibility, and endurance. Most organizations recommend at least 30 minutes of physical activity for a minimum of three days per week at a pace that will raise your heartbeat and breath rate, but you should be doing some type of exercise at least five or more days of the week. For weight reduction you may need to increase your time commitment spent on exercise.

Some aerobic activities include brisk walking outdoors, treadmill walking, step-type exercises where you climb stairs, play tennis, jog, swim, do aqua aerobics, take step or aerobic exercise classes, Pilates, and/or use elliptical machines. One recommendation is to purchase a pedometer at your local sporting goods store so you can clip it onto your belt and then begin walking. This device measures your steps to determine the distance you have walked or jogged as well as the calories burned. Most exercise experts recommend that you take at least 10,000 steps per day.

A pedometer makes most women more conscious of their exercise and helps them to make decisions to increase the number of steps each day. Walking farther and at a faster pace to the office or shopping, skipping the cab to walk extra city blocks, choosing the stairs instead of the elevator, going for a walk during coffee breaks or after meals are a few creative ways to add more exercise to your daily routine.

Most exercise plans consist of three stages: a warm up period of gentle stretching postures, an aerobic set of exercises that speeds up your heart and respiration, and cool down exercises. Slow, gentle stretching prepares your muscles for the more strenuous activity to come by increasing your blood flow. These exercises also help increase your range of motion (flexibility) and stability (balance). They shift you from being in a quiet resting state to warming up your entire body. Moving into aerobic exercises is where you use many different muscles repeatedly, which ultimately strengthens your heart and lungs. Your heart rate increases and you are sweating while burning calories. During the cool down period, your exercises are slower and have fewer repetitions. Your heart rate slowly returns to baseline as you begin to relax from the vigorous exercises you have just completed. Finally, you are ready to stop and rest.

In order to gain the effects of exercise, the American Heart Association recommends aerobic exercise 20 to 30 minutes at least three to four times per week. The more you do, the better your health will be. Some other organizations advocate up to six times per week! Maintaining an active, healthy, vibrant lifestyle throughout the whole week will help you feel better, gain strength, and maintain excellent health during survivorship.

Some basic steps you should take before beginning your exercise plan include assessing your present level of fitness, flexibility, and muscle strength. Discuss your fitness goals with your physician and make certain they are realistic and obtainable before starting a program. Choosing lofty goals only sets you up for failure and disappointment. Consider the time needed to invest in the activity, and the cost (if any) of the program that you wish to implement. Make certain you have the correct clothing and footware before starting your exercises.

Monitoring your progress is also another important facet for any exercise schedule. Some fitness experts advise people to keep an exercise diary or log book to document their workouts and how they feel afterwards. Listing the specifics enables you to reference them at a later date. An exercise diary can record the date, type of activity, time spent, calories burned, and the level of intensity. It's fun to review it over time to track your fitness progress.

If you believe that you are a novice when it comes to exercise and the discipline it takes to stick with a plan, then consider joining your local sports club, YMCA, or YWCA. There may be fitness centers located close to your home or place of employment. Choose one that is convenient and fits your budget. Many offer organized fitness classes like **yoga**, aerobics, or Pilates. Many gyms have credentialed fitness instructors (trainers) who can be invaluable assets for designing exercise programs and individualized lessons that meet your personal goals. They also offer instruction on how to use the weight and cardiovascular machines correctly to prevent injury and muscle damage. Before choosing an instructor, verify his or her credentials and training to make certain they are aware of your underlying medical conditions that will influence your exercise plan.

Yoga

a type of exercise where the emphasis is on long, slow stretching into various postures, and using slow, deep breathing to hold the posture. It is said to unify the elements of mind and body to help eliminate stress and decrease fatigue.

I decided that even if I went to the gym and laid down on the treadmill, I was getting my behind in there. People think cancer patients always lose weight. Wrong! If you're having chemo and all you feel like eating is macaroni and cheese, guess what? I upped my training sessions to three days a week—a luxury not all budgets or schedules allow, I realize, but that is no excuse for doing nothing. A structured program where something or someone compels you to show up is best, no doubt, but anything is better than nothing. The hardest thing about exercising is beginning. Put on those sneakers and walk out the door. Even if you just go around the block, good! Bet you'll go further, though. I came to see exercise as essential not just to my overall recovery and fitness, but to my confidence, energy, and sense of well-being. All this stuff is scientifically documented, of course, but I'm telling you, it's the best thing you can do for yourself. It makes everything better. Go at your own pace and do what you can. You will amaze yourself. And you know what, dur-

ing treatment I definitely had some days that were better than others, but I never did lie down on that treadmill.

Frances S.

39. How can I identify and overcome my resistance to a more active lifestyle?

Despite that the health benefits of exercise are well known, the majority of North American women fail to exercise on a daily basis. Family, friends, co-workers, and the community in which we live can greatly affect our ability to exercise. It is no wonder that many of us create obstacles that prevent us from enjoying an active exercise program.

If your friends are fitness gurus, you are more likely to enjoy active events with them, but if you come from a long line of couch potatoes, then you are more likely to be sedentary. If you live far from the town recreational center or do not have a park nearby, it is tempting to avoid exercising. The Center for Disease Control and Prevention in Atlanta has a program entitled, "Active Community Environments Initiative," which promotes the awareness and development of locations where all people can enjoy activities like walking, running, and active recreation. Your physical activity can take place throughout your environment. The local park or recreational center, sidewalks or park trails, even walking around the local shopping mall offers opportunities to exercise in all types of weather. Some schools allow the public to walk their track after hours or on their campus. Those living in more rural areas can find neighborhoods, meadows, deer trails, and quiet roads to hike. All it takes is a little creativity to find a new and exciting place to exercise. Use your imagination!

According to Sallis and Hovel's 1990 article, "Determinants of Exercise Behavior," which appeared in the *Exercise and Sports Science Review*, and Sallis et al.'s, "Predictors of Adoption and Maintenance of Vigorous Physical Activity in Men and Women," published in *Preventative Medicine*, some of the personal barriers to starting and continuing an exercise plan include lack of self-motivation, boredom with routine, simply not finding exercise enjoyable or fun, lack of time, and finding exercise inconvenient. Fear of injury, lack of management skills to set goals and monitor progress, and lack of encouragement from family and friends are other barriers.

Practical suggestions for maintaining an exercise plan include identifying and committing specific time slots for when you exercise each day and monitoring your progress. Choose to make exercise a part of your daily routine. Skip the shuttle bus and walk or ride your bicycle to work. Take the dog for several daily walks each day or park your vehicle in the furthest spot in the mall and walk to the entrance at the opposite side of the building. Invite a friend or work partner to join you in your exercise. Exercise often becomes a social event. Try new activities that you have never done before but have always wanted to try! Learn a new sport. Canoeing, kayaking, skiing, skating, and ballroom dancing can be fun. Join a softball team. Let your imagination be your guide.

By joining your local YMCA, YWCA, or community health club, you will meet new people who also enjoy active lifestyles. If you feel tired or bored, plan a different exercise to do or route to walk. Read a book, watch television, listen to music, or even read the newspaper while doing light exercise, such as cycling on a stationary bicycle or walking the treadmill.

Be sure to stretch before and after your vigorous exercise plan to warm up and cool down your muscles. Be aware of your fitness level and try to increase the intensity of your exercises gradually. In foul weather, have a list of indoor activities that you enjoy doing, such as indoor swimming and aerobic exercises at the health spa, indoor tennis, or dancing. For those with children, plan activities that the whole family can enjoy. Go hiking in the mountains, or plan a beach picnic after a day of swimming in the surf. Pile the babies into the stroller and go for a long walk. Cycle together. If you travel frequently for work, make certain the hotel you are staying at has a health club or pack a skipping rope or resistance band in your bag. Go exploring on foot in the new city for an hour a day. You will learn much about the new destination and in the process burn a lot of calories!

40. What exercises can I do?

Some people find it difficult to stick with an exercise plan. One answer for some people is to have an exercise buddy (spouse, other family member, or friend) to help motivate them to keep on their physical fitness plan. Others feel that varying the aerobic activities helps prevent boredom. Variety is often the spice that some people need in order to maintain an exercise plan. On some days listen to music and other days read a book while exercising. Make exercising fun by reading, watching television, or chatting with your workout partner. On other days, skip the gym and head outdoors with the dog for a long walk along the beach.

Exercise

Sometimes group activities can replace individual workouts. Check out the local media for community neighborhood clean up days, gallery walks, sporting events, and other activities that are opportunities to get physical. Look into your local sports club to see if their activities are interesting. Sometimes varying the time of day you work out is helpful and relieves the routine or helps with scheduling conflicts. You do not need to spend a lot of money on health clubs or buy fancy sports equipment to maintain a fitness program. On the other hand, some people find that joining a health club provides them the incentive to continue to regularly participate in physical fitness. Walking is an inexpensive way to start any exercise program. All you need is a pair of good, supportive running shoes.

Tables 1 and 2 list a few physical activities recommended by to the Center for Disease Control and Pre-

Table 1   Moderate Activities

Walking at a moderate or brisk pace	Hiking	Stationary bicycle using moderate effort
Water aerobics	Yoga	Animal care
Gymnastics	Jumping on a trampoline	Rowing a boat or using a row machine
Weight training using universal machines, dumbbells, rowing, and/or cables	Boxing-punching bag	Ballroom dancing
	Disco dancing	Modern and jazz dancing
	Tennis doubles	Golfing, wheeling or carrying your clubs
Square dancing	Basketball, shooting baskets	Volleyball
Ballet	Curling	Juggling
Softball	Archery	Downhill skiing or snowmobiling
Frisbee or baton twirling	Waterskiing or sailing	Canoeing or rafting
Badminton	Deer hunting	Horseback riding
Swimming	Gardening in the yard	Light snow shoveling
Fishing	Aqua aerobics	Line dancing
Skateboarding	Kayaking	Fencing
Moderate housework: scrubbing the floor		
Snorkeling		

Table 2　More Strenuous Activities

Aerobic dancing	Jogging, hiking	Backpacking
Fast step-type dancing, like salsa and hustle	Step aerobics	Karate, judo
	Stair climbing	Circuit weight training
Jumping jacks	Soccer	Boxing in the ring
Clogging	Lacrosse	Field hockey
Rugby	Squash	Sledding, tobogganing
Racquet ball	Skipping	Playing ice hockey
Running	Jumping rope	Shoveling heavy snow
Playing polo	Moving heavy furniture	Walking with 50 pounds
Pushing a non-motorized lawn mower	Running up a flight of stairs	or more
Vigorous play with children		Brisk walking (more than 4 miles per hour)

Source: U.S. Department of Health and Human Services, Public Health Service, Center for Disease Control and Prevention, National Center for Chronic Disease Prevention and Health Promotion, Division of Nutrition and Physical Activity. *Promoting Physical Activity: A Guide for Community Action.* Champaign, IL: Human Kinetics; 1999. (Table adapted from Ainsworth BE, Haskell WL, Leon AS, et al. Compendium of physical activities: classification of energy costs of human physical activities. *Medicine and Science in Sports and Exercise* 1993;25:71–80.

vention (CDC) and ACSM Guidelines that can be incorporated into your exercise plan.

41. How do I avoid injury or hurting myself during exercise?

If you never had an exercise plan (that is, you do a minimum of 30 minutes of strenuous exercise several days per week), have been out of the exercise world for over a year, or have some medical or chronic illness(es), it is always best to consult your doctor.

Provide your doctor with a complete history and physical examination before starting on any exercise plan. Discuss any issues of starting an exercise plan with your doctor, as he or she may suggest limitations as to the types and force of a particular exercise you want to begin. Tell your doctor the types and dosages of your medications and ask if there are any reasons why you should not (contraindications) begin a regimen of physical exercise. Discuss the amount and type of exercise, the activities and the intensity, as well as the times of the day you plan to exercise. In particular, it is important to check with your doctor about vigorous exercise activities such as weightlifting, working out on weight machines, jogging, and swimming. Be sure to get a list of activities that, given your cancer history, you should avoid because of your unique medical history. You should always try to gradually increase the amount of exercise you are doing, especially if you have not exercised for a long time. Make sure you have eaten, are well hydrated (see Question 32 about water intake), and are wearing the appropriate sportswear for your activity.

Please remember that if you have any shortness of breath, chest pain, dizziness, feel light-headed, or experience discomfort, it is important that you always stop your exercises and consult your physician immediately. Pressure in your chest, arms, or jaw discomfort should also alert you to seek immediate medical attention. If you are tired, don't overexert yourself. Always listen to the signs and symptoms you are getting from your body and rest when needed.

PART 5

Pain and Sleep Management

What can I do to alleviate my fatigue?

How is cancer pain treated?

How can I improve the duration and quality of my sleep patterns?

More ...

PAIN MANAGEMENT

42. I feel so tired all of the time. What can I do to decrease my fatigue?

Fatigue is a common problem for those who have undergone cancer and its treatments. Feeling tired and listless is devastating because it directly impacts on your daily activities as well the lives of others in your household and your extended circle of family and friends. Most of those with cancer and many survivors feel a general lack of energy, body malaise, and have a difficult time concentrating.

Some of the more common causes of fatigue include: side effects of medications, underactive thyroid gland, destruction of cancer cells, infection, uncontrolled pain, fever, poor nutrition, and a reduced number of red blood cells (**anemia**). Other factors that influence tiredness may include mental depression, poor sleeping patterns, anxiety, and emotional stress.

Anemia

a condition in which the number of red blood cells is below normal.

It is always important to discuss your concerns with your healthcare team. Some causes of fatigue are easily treated. Before your visit to the clinic, describe (quantify) and record the times of the day when you feel most tired. Certain medications like epoietin (Procrit®, Epogen®) or darbepoetin (Aranesep®) can be given by injection to women who have anemia, and these medications have been shown to help with fatigue. According to Memorial Sloan Kettering's recent handout on fatigue management, other helpful techniques to decrease fatigue include:

- *Practice good sleep patterns.* Sleep extra hours, go to bed earlier, or stay in bed later in the morning (see

Question 47). If you are unable to sleep or believe you suffer from insomnia, you may benefit from a short course of sleep medications. Ask your doctor if these are appropriate in your situation. Most prescriptions are for a short time because they can be habit-forming.

- Eliminate difficult activities that cause fatigue (those that drain your energy) and pace yourself throughout the day.
- Schedule rest throughout the day by taking short naps.
- Ask for help from family and friends. Getting help with some of the activities of daily living helps you to be less tired and others to feel good about themselves because they are doing something tangible to help you. Household chores like cooking, cleaning, and grocery shopping can be delegated to family or friends. Child care can also be delegated.
- Do not be afraid to limit your activities and obligations. Learn to say "no" but do not isolate yourself from your social network.
- Ask your healthcare team if some of the medications you are taking may be contributing to your lack of energy and fatigue. If so, then discuss a substitute medication or whether you can limit your intake.
- Plan a well balanced diet, eat plenty of fruits and vegetables, and drink lots of fluids (8 to 10 glasses of water per day). Avoid caffeinated beverages or alcohol, especially in the evening hours. See a nutritionist or consider incorporating some vitamin supplements (see Questions 33–36).
- Maintain a light exercise plan that is tailored to your needs. Exercise actually boosts your energy level as long as you do not overdo it (see Questions 37–41). Start slowly with an easy exercise such as walking, and then gradually build up your stamina

by increasing your walking distance as your fatigue lessens. Maintain a good balance between mild exercise and periods of rest.

- Plan special or important activities when you know your strength will be at its highest level.
- Try new activities that promote relaxation. Yoga, **meditation**, and Tai Chi are all excellent choices.
- Listen to your favorite soothing music before bedtime and avoid excessive stimulating activities before naps and bedtime.
- If you are feeling anxious or depressed, ask for professional help. Peer support groups are located all over North America (contact the American Cancer Society).
- Spiritual and religious connections can soothe and uplift the human spirit. Talking with someone in your religious institution may bring you a sense of tranquility, which alleviates fatigue. Reading books about your faith, watching spiritually enlightening movies, and attending classes, discussion groups, or spending time with others in your spiritual circle may help you tap into a deeper connection with yourself and enrich your spirituality.
- Stop and sit frequently when you are tired.

Consider using a cane, walker, wheelchair, or scooter if mobility is an issue. Use grab bars in bathrooms, sit down when getting dressed or putting on makeup, or allow yourself to hold onto the arm of your spouse, family member, or friend to keep steady while walking.

Excellent information about managing fatigue is on the Internet. Contact the Oncology Nursing Society (http://www.cancersymptoms.org/fatigue) or the National

Meditation

ancient techniques using deep, slow breathing to calm the mind and help the body relax; often used in conjunction with visualization.

Comprehensive Cancer Network (http://www.nccn. org) for more information.

43. Why should I control my cancer pain?

Living in constant chronic pain can be very distressing and negatively affect your quality of life. Activities of your daily living as well as your overall mental, physical, and emotional well being are impacted. Many cancer patients believe—unjustly—that they need to suffer in silence. However, be assured that most cancer pain can be effectively controlled. This means that you can enjoy life again, sleep better, and eat more healthily once your pain is under some type of control.

By controlling your discomfort, you can effectively regain control of your life, enjoy a more active vibrant lifestyle, and enjoy social connections. Letting your pain get out of control often leads to feelings of anger, frustration, depression, or even isolation and stress.

Controlling your pain often involves a variety of professionals, which may include your cancer (oncology) doctors, nurses, pharmacists, anesthesiologists, neurologists, and perhaps a specialist in pain management. There is no reasonable rationale to suffer in silence, be stoic or brave, believe that discussing your pain or discomfort is a sign of weakness, or to even rationalize your suffering as being part of the healing process. Discuss your concerns with your healthcare team. They can not treat your pain problem if they do not know that one exists.

One reason why some patients fail to discuss pain control is the false notion that if they do take prescribed pain medications they will become addicted. This is rarely the case even if you are taking strong medications like narcotics or opioids. Some people fear the potential side effects of the medications, like constipation, nausea and vomiting, lightheadedness, feeling confused, or even a feeling of loss of control. Discuss your personal concerns with your doctor so that your dosing schedule can be modified or medications changed to minimize side effects while maximizing your control of pain.

There are many types of cancer pain, including acute, chronic, and breakthrough pain. Pain can come from the cancer tumor itself or be a result of the surgery, chemotherapy, or radiation therapy you have received. **Phantom pain** can occur at the site of an amputation or limb removal, and some women who have had mastectomies or complete breast removal can feel abnormal pain, sensations, or discomfort at the area where the breast is missing.

I'm one of those people who "hates to take things" like pain or sleep medications. And that is ridiculous. I've finally come to realize I want my body's energy to HEAL and not to struggle with pain or insomnia. I know when I need them and when I don't, and so will you. I think of these medicines as working with my body, and that's what we want.

Frances S.

44. How is cancer pain treated?

Sometimes cancer pain treatment will involve medications and non-medical techniques that can minimize your pain. You may be prescribed some medication and may also find it helpful to use some of the non-medication techniques as well for the management of

Phantom pain

a type of painful sensation that can occur at the site of an amputation or limb removal; some women who have had mastectomies or complete breast removal can feel abnormal pain, sensations, or discomfort at the area where the breast is missing.

your pain. It may be helpful to develop and implement an adequate pain management plan with your health-care team.

Keeping a diary where you document your pain levels and quality throughout the day can be helpful. Try to document the intensity on a scale from one to ten, where ten is the worst pain ever experienced and one or zero is pain-free. Mark down the type of pain. Does it feel dull? Throbbing? Sharp? Does it come and go or is it constant? Are there things you do that make your pain better or worse? Also keep record of how your pain is managed. This would be your medication and other techniques you may use to control your pain.

45. What are the common pain medications?

Some pain medication is over-the-counter, where you can buy it at a store and others are prescribed by your medical doctor. Before your medical visit, it is important to write a list (or bring) all of the medications you are taking. These drugs can be analyzed so that possible side effects or drug interactions can be minimized.

According to the American Cancer Society's guide on pain management, the following are very important questions to ask your physician before taking some pain medications.

- How much medication should I take? What is the dose?
- What is the recommended dosing schedule? (How often should I take it?)
- Can I take more if I am still in pain? How long should I wait before it activates? If I can take more,

how much? If no, then how long do I have to wait before the next dose?

- Should I take the medication with food or on an empty stomach?
- Can I drink alcohol with this medication? Are there foods to avoid?
- Can I work, drive, or operate machinery on this medication?
- How does this medication interact with the other medications I am already taking?
- What are the common side effects from this type of medication? How can I prevent or treat them?
- Does this medication interact with certain foods, herbs, or vitamins?
- What do I do if I run out of my prescription? What is your office practice for renewing medications?
- Is this covered by my insurance? Can I take a less expensive generic form?

Some of the medications typically used for pain control are listed below. This list is not exhaustive and new mediations may be offered by your doctor. Pain medications can come in the form of pills (taken by mouth), patches that attach to your skin, in liquid (elixir) form, or they may be injected into your bloodstream (intravenous), muscle (intramuscular), or into space around nerve endings in your spine (epidural). Suppositories also may be used.

Non-opioids. Acetaminophen, aspirin, ibuprofen, and other nonsteroidal anti-inflammatory (NSAIDs) drugs fit into this category. Gastrointestinal upset can occur with the NSAIDs. Some are over-the-counter (can be purchase at your local pharmacy) without a prescription. Stronger doses of these types of medications may require a doctor's prescription.

Opioids. This category includes morphine, fentanyl, demerol, codeine, and oxycodone. Some of the more likely side effects of the opioids include drowsiness, constipation, nausea, or vomiting. Some people may experience itchiness over their body or mental changes like confusion or hallucinations. Opioids can be addictive. When you no longer need opioids for pain control, you should be weaned off this medication slowly over time. Gradually diminishing your dose and times of taking this type of medication avoids the rapid withdrawal symptoms, which include generally feeling bad, a flu-like syndrome, disturbed sleep, preoccupation with physical symptoms, and a lower threshold for tolerating stress. These symptoms may go away in a short period of time in healthy individuals.

Antidepressants and Anticonvulsants. These can be used for nerve pain or pain that causes burning or tingling. Antidepressants have the added benefit of treating mood disorders as well as chronic pain syndromes. Some common side effects of these drugs are dry-mouth, drop in blood pressure, an inability to urinate, or drowsiness.

Delaying treatment with medications or "holding off" between doses is also not effective in controlling your pain (see Question 43). In fact, it is counterproductive to your overall comfort and sense of pain relief. Taking your medications on a fixed timetable may be the best method to effectively control your cancer pain and distress. It is important to remember that if you experience any side effects or complications from your medications, seek professional medical advice. Your physician can tell you the best method to manage these upsetting and bothersome side effects or even change your medication to another that provides you with more comfort.

46. Are there non-medication ways to control my cancer pain?

You can use a number of strategies to cope with your pain and anxiety. Some include relaxation techniques such as **hypnosis**, biofeedback, **guided imagery**, **acupuncture**, deep rhythmic breathing, or physical therapy. Many comprehensive cancer institutions have an integrative medicine division, a department of alternative or complementary medicine, or have resources where these services can be provided.

If you suffer from chronic pain and are having difficulty adjusting to this aspect of your survivorship, it may be helpful to seek some emotional counseling or supportive care. Many healthcare professionals are specifically trained in pain management for the cancer survivor and can help you to control your emotional and physical discomfort. Questions 60–72 discuss a range of specialized techniques like reflexology, Shiatsu massage, aromatherapy, **Reiki**, meditation, and yoga.

SLEEP

47. How can I improve my sleep patterns?

According to the National Commission on Sleep Disorders Research, over 40 million Americans suffer from some type of sleep disturbance. Sleep disturbance is defined as **insomnia** (inability to fall asleep and remain asleep throughout the night), sleep apnea (stopping breathing during sleep leading to poor quality of sleep and not feeling refreshed in the morning), narcolepsy (immediate and unprovoked falling asleep), **hypersomnia** (sleeping too much), or restless leg syndrome. Many women report increased insomnia, sleep apnea, and poor sleep patterns immediately before or during the menopause transition. Hot flashes may be a significant contributor to poor sleep quality; however, other medical issues such as underlying illnesses also may play an important role in sleep problems for women.

Insomnia
lack of sleep.

Hypersomnia
sleeping all of the time.

Most people are chronically fatigued because we rarely allow ourselves sufficient rest for our body and mind to recover from our busy and hectic activities each day. Many women feel exhausted by the end of the day only to find that there are yet more chores or activities to be done before they can rest. Over-worked and over-scheduling combined with poor sleep habits cause a life of exhaustion and fatigue.

Sleeping well at night can help you feel better and refreshed and may boost your energy level. You will be more alert and have more zip for life's activities. If you have trouble sleeping through the night, or if you feel that the quality of your sleep leaves you still feeling tired, try these suggestions.

At bedtime:

- Go to bed at the same time each evening and get up at the same time in the morning. Establish a nightly routine and stick with it as much as possible. Your body needs predictability.

- Keep the temperature in your bedroom comfortable. Hot flashes can interrupt sleep and upset your ability to be rested even if they do not awaken you during the night. Hot flashes of menopause can influence your feelings of restfulness and disturb a deep, restful sleep.
- Keep the bedroom quiet and dark when you are sleeping. If noise is a problem, try earplugs or background or "white" noise such as a CD with ocean sounds or raindrops. If cannot make your bedroom dark, wear a sleep mask. Unplug your telephone, disconnect your cellular mobile phone, and shut down your home or work computer and Blackberry.
- Do not let pets sleep in your bedroom. They are often "bed hogs" and can move around, thereby interrupting your sleep.
- Create a bedtime routine of things you do to slow down from your day. Play cards, read, or enjoy other quiet activities immediately before you go to bed. Most sleep experts' advise that you not watch television or use the Internet before bed as these activities may be too stimulating.
- Use your bed only for sleep and sex. Create a loving, tranquil environment. Purchase new, comfortable sheets and linens. Try a nice feathery pillow cover!
- Take only your own prescription medications and use them as directed. Take any prescribed sleeping pill(s) 40 to 60 minutes before bedtime, so they have time to work before you get into bed. Some fast-acting medications must be taken right before going into bed. Consult with your healthcare professional if you think you may need a prescription sleep aid.
- Use a relaxation exercise just before going to sleep. Try muscle relaxation (where you tense and relax each muscle from the bottom of your feet to the top

of your head while lying face up), mental imagery, massage by your partner, a warm bath, listening to calm music or a soothing classical symphony, or even a few minutes of light reading.

- Do not eat a heavy fatty meal before going to bed. Limit your fluids before going to bed, especially if you must get up at night to urinate.

- Avoid caffeinated beverages, nicotine, and alcohol in the late afternoon and several hours before bedtime. All can keep you awake and interfere with sleep. Try drinking decaffeinated herbal teas that are calming such as passionflower, a combination of herbs for sleepiness, or chamomile.

- If you can not fall asleep within a reasonable time, get out of bed and do something relaxing. Continue reading your book or listen to more music. Staying in bed will frustrate you and can get you more upset.

- Try keeping a sleep diary where you record your sleep patterns. This could be the time you go to bed, what you did before sleeping, naps, and whether you wake up during the night. It is also essential to document how you feel in the morning. You should bring this booklet to your healthcare provider who may use this information to establish a diagnosis of a sleep disorder.

- If you can not get your mind away from your worries, get up and make a list of the things you are worried about. List things you can do to decrease or eliminate that worry (e.g., ask the doctor about a symptom, discuss your fears with a friend or your partner). Organize your calendar for the next day. Sometimes just writing things down on paper helps soften your feelings of life being out of control. Then you can release your inner demand that they must be done immediately and understand that you will do them tomorrow, next week, or whenever.

Practical suggestions of things to do during the day are:

- Exercise each day, but not before bedtime. Any form of exercise is acceptable.
- Keep a sleep diary to share with your doctor. Your healthcare clinician may be able to offer suggestions or prescribe a sleep aid.
- Do not take naps.

PART 6

Symptoms and Management of Menopause

How can I manage my hot flashes?

Should I take hormone replacement therapy?

What can I do to maintain vaginal health during menopause?

What are Kegel exercises?

More . . .

The strict definition of menopause is that a woman does not have a menstrual cycle for one year. A woman may go through *natural menopause*, where her cycles stop spontaneously, usually around age 51. *Chemical menopause* occurs when the woman has received chemicals (like chemotherapy) or medications that temporarily or permanently stop her cycles. A woman may receive some prescribed medications, such as a gonadotropin releasing hormone (GnRH) agonist, which shuts down her pituitary gland and ovaries, thereby creating a menopausal state. *Surgical menopause* is when both ovaries are removed so hormones are no longer produced.

48. What is a hot flash?

The exact reason and cause for hot flashes is not yet known. However, some menopausal research scientists believe that a hormone called luteinizing hormone (LH) is released at the same time as the levels of estrogen decrease. This release of LH may contribute to a change in certain nerve pathways and ultimately lead to veins getting larger for no apparent reason. This reaction can cause skin flushing (change of skin color to red), increased perspiration, and sudden changes in blood flow, body temperature, and heart rate. Hot flashes can make you feel as if you are fully dressed in a sauna. Your internal thermostat suddenly increases to 110°F and your face suddenly flushes hot and red. You begin to perspire profusely.

Hot flashes can usually begin as a sensation of pressure or warm heat in the head, neck, chest, and back, which spreads to the entire body. They can begin several years before menses stops completely in the perimenopausal period (transition years). The number of and length of time of a hot flash are different for each woman: Some woman may experience as few as one a day or as many as three an hour, when others may not experience any hot flashes at all. Hot flashes usually interrupt sleep, which may result in feelings of irritability and a condition of sleeplessness called insomnia (see Question 47). The good news is that the number of hot flashes usually decreases as you get further on in your menopause.

Many women experience hot flashes that are not troublesome and do not warrant therapy. Others are debilitated by their menopausal syndrome. Quality of life issues are paramount and many women seek therapies for their hot flashes. Hormonal therapy with estrogen and/or progesterone therapy and other therapies are readily available. Consult with your clinician about your symptoms.

49. Can I take hormone therapy?

Hormone therapy (HT) has gotten a lot of negative media press since the publication of the Women's Health Initiative (WHI) Study, which linked estrogen and progesterone use for menopausal symptoms with a slightly increased risk for heart attacks, breast cancer, and strokes. As a result of this widely publicized study, many women stopped taking their hormonal pills. According to the American Medical Association, only about 7.6 million women used hormones in 2004 when in 2002 there were close to 18.5 million users. Unfortunately, those women who were on estrogen alone because of having had a hysterectomy also decreased the amount of pills they took as well. Women with an intact uterus also need a progestin/progesterone compound to help reduce the risk for uterine cancer.

Although many women are appropriate candidates for **hormone replacement therapy (HRT),** many stop or fail to start the medications that can be very helpful for their general feelings of well being. Hormonal therapy is now no longer advocated for the primary prevention of cardiovascular disease; however, it still remains an effective treatment for vaginal dryness and hot flashes. There are many low-dose preparations including the patch, rings, gels, vaginal tablets, creams, and other formulations, which should be used in the lowest doses for the shortest amount of time for menopausal symptom relief. Every woman should carefully educate herself and analyze the risks and benefits of taking hormones, especially with regard to their symptoms and family and personal history. It is important to discuss your concerns regarding estrogen and progesterone hormones with your gynecologist. In fact, many women are appropriate candidates for short-term use of these medications.

If you do decide to take hormones to help with hot flashes and other menopausal complaints, be sure to see your healthcare provider annually for a physical examination, clinical breast examination, and annual mammogram. Breast self-examination and a risk assessment should also be done on a regular basis. If your relatives develop cancers, discuss your continuation on the hormones with your doctor. Side effects of hormonal therapy can be minimal but it is important to report any abnormal symptoms (like vaginal bleeding) to your doctor. Lower dosage products can be tai-

Hormone replacement therapy (HRT)

estrogen and progesterone that can be given in various combinations to relieve the symptoms of menopause. When estrogen is given alone it is called estrogen replacement.

lored to your specific medical needs and should relieve your symptoms while minimizing side effects.

50. What are bioidentical hormones? Are they safe?

According to the American College of Obstetricians and Gynecologists committee opinion, compounded bioidentical hormones are plant-derived hormones that are created, mixed, and packaged by a pharmacist who can customize the product according to the physician's specifications. Most compounded products have not undergone strict scientific study and there may be concerns about safety, purity, and efficacy of these products.

Compounded products have the same risks as conventional pharmacologically produced hormones. It is also important to know that there is no medically recognized governing organization like the FDA that officially regulates compounding substances. The most common compounded hormones include: dehydroepiandrosterone, pregnenolone, testosterone, progesterone, estrone, estradiol, and estriol. They often come in a variety of routes of administration including oral, sublingual, implants, injectables, or suppositories. Biest® is a common bioidentical estrogen consisting of 20% estradiol and 80% estriol. Another, Triest®, contains 10% estradiol, 10% estrone, and 80% estriol. Sometimes insurance companies will not reimburse for these compounded products, so they can be expensive for the individual. The Food and Drug Administration does not regulate these products and there is growing concern within the medical community about their purity, safety, and efficacy. Many do not contain the same amount of concentrated active ingredient claimed on their packaging. No scientific data support the claim that bioidentical hormones are safer than conventional prescribed hormonal therapy with respect to health or cancer concerns.

Salivary oral testing of hormones is often advocated by those who use bioidentical hormones. Some claim that the salivary hormone results can be used to tailor an individual preparation for a woman and her unique hormonal needs. Unfortunately, there is no medical evidence that salivary hormones provide any clinically useful information. Salivary hormones depend on a multitude of factors, including the particular hormone tested and the time of day the test was conducted. There is also concern that there may not be a direct correlation between salivary hormones and biologically-active hormone levels, clinical state, or therapeutic results. The fact exists that there is large variation of levels within the same individual and between individuals. If you are considering taking bioidentical hormones or are now taking a prescribed compound, know that it may be dangerous. It is strongly recommended that you discuss the risks of bioidentical hormones with your cancer specialist.

51. I do not want to take hormones. How can I manage my hot flashes?

Even though many women may be candidates for estrogen alone or a combination of estrogen and progesterone therapies, they may choose not to use these products because of personal choice or fear of developing breast cancer or another type of hormonally sensitive cancer. Some breast cancer survivors may decline systemic hormonal use with estrogen and progesterone because they may believe that these hormones may trigger the regrowth of a tumor, or stimulate a preexisting cancer in the breast. There is fear that these hormones can stimulate a recurrence or the development of another primary breast cancer in a woman already deemed at risk.

There are other ways to help minimize some of the adverse effects of hot flashes. Some useful techniques are:

1. Wear absorbent cotton clothing or dress in layers so that the outermost layers can be removed when you get a hot flash. Cotton is a preferred fabric because it is quick drying; its wicking effect traps and removes moisture from your body. Special sleepwear has been developed for those with nighttime hot flashes (Wicking Menopause pajamas®).

2. As soon as you feel a hot flash is coming on, drink an ice-cold glass of water or put a cold compress on your face. Misting type bottles can help you spritz water. Relief may also be felt from running cold water on your wrists or immersing your feet in cold water.

3. Lowering the thermostat will help you maintain some control and help save money on your heating bill. Turn down the heat in the winter and raise the air-conditioning in the summer. It is easy for your partner to put on a sweater or sleep with a heavier blanket.

4. Use a room fan near places where you habitually sit or wave a hand-held fan. Fancy paper or fabric fans make beautiful accessories to any stylish outfit. Keep one in your purse and another in your car or office for easy access.

5. Biofeedback techniques and relaxation techniques like yoga, meditation, and Tai Chi may be helpful for troublesome hot flashes (see Questions 60–72). These activities also are helpful in decreasing stress and anxiety.

6. Research has shown that women who exercise regularly may have less difficulty with menopausal hot flashes (see Questions 37 and 38). Start an exercise program today.

7. Avoid cigarette smoking.

8. Sleep near an open window.

9. Change sleeping attire and bed linen to lighter fabrics.

Chillow

a personal cooling pillow that may help with sleep. It works by keeping your head cool.

10. Purchase a personal cooling pillow (**Chillow®**) to help you sleep more comfortably. It works by keeping your head cool. Visit the Web site www.chillow.com!

11. Keep a hot flash diary. Record the number of hot flashes each day and quantify their intensity. Show your diary to your clinician.

12. Avoid hot baths or showers in the two hours prior to going to bed.

13. Practice the paced respiration techniques described below.

The way that you breathe has been shown to reduce the frequency and intensity of menopausal hot flashes. Studies show that when the paced respiration technique is used correctly, it can ease hot flashes by at least 50%.

Two steps to do the paced respiration:

1. Make a conscious effort to remain calm. In a relaxed manner, take six to eight slow, deep breaths through your nose. Each cycle of breath (in and out) should take at least a minute.

2. During each inhalation, allow the air to slowly enter your body, filling your abdomen first, and then your lungs, filling your body with more and more air. If you place your hand on your belly, you can feel your abdomen expand and sense your chest cavity as it widens. Exhale through your nose or mouth just as slowly and evenly, feeling your chest and abdomen as they contract, sending all of the air out.

You should practice these paced respirations for at least fifteen minutes at least two times every day. This breathing exercise also can be done anytime day or night in addition to the two times recommended. In addition to doing this exercise while you are experiencing a hot flash, it is very useful to do these breaths while waiting in the grocery store line, driving in traffic, or when you are in any type of stressful situation. You also may find that paced respirations are helpful to do in situations where in the past you have had a hot flash (e.g., being in a room that feels too warm). Paced respirations may also act to calm your mind and lessen distress and anxiety (Adapted from Memorial Sloan-Kettering Cancer Center patient educational materials).

I've acquired a lovely little collection of fans (none of them antique or expensive, by the way) and have found them very handy. Portable and practical, they are also quite a lot of fun and almost always conversation pieces. Not to mention fashion accessories.

Frances S.

52. Can modifying my diet help with my hot flashes?

A healthy diet for the menopausal female is important for overall general health, fitness, and strength. Many women find some relief in menopausal hot flashes with some minor dietary changes and/or the addition of some basic vitamin and mineral supplements. Moderation is the key when making any changes to your food intake.

There are some practical suggestions that have proven helpful in some women. Try one or all of them to help reduce the number or intensity of the hot flashes.

Avoid certain triggers that may include caffeine, alcohol (including beer, wine; and liquor), and spicy foods. Consider adding some vitamin supplements such as vitamin B_6 (200 or 250 mg daily) *OR* Peridin C (two tablets three times a day). These may help. Start with the above over-the-counter medicines and allow at least four to six weeks for them to work. If possible, add one supplement at a time so that you can determine if it is working for you.

53. Can complementary therapies and alternative medicines be used to manage severe, debilitating hot flashes?

Complementary medicine and alternative techniques or therapies often utilize the disciplines of modern science and medicine and couples them with ancient philosophies from different cultures. As a result, many techniques incorporate modern Western and traditional Eastern philosophies. Many strategies have gained popularity as they can help ease suffering and promote healing or feelings of well being.

At some point or another, many cancer survivors will consider using a variety of herbal supplements or other unconventional techniques to help maintain an improved quality of life or minimize troublesome side effects. Doubtless, many women may choose alternative herbs and other techniques to help manage their severe and debilitating hot flashes. Some of the more common herbal preparations that some menopausal women have tried in order to help control hot flashes include: isoflavones, black cohosh, chaste tree berry, ginseng, dong quai, evening primrose oil, wild yam, mother wort, red clover, linden flower, yarrow, and green tea extract.

The American College of Obstetricians and Gynecologists Task Force on Hormone Therapy has examined the scientific evidence for soy, black cohosh, red clover, and Mexican progesterone yam cream for the treatment of menopausal hot flashes. Unfortunately, these products did not reduce hot flashes to a clinically significant amount. Still, many perimenopasual and menopausal women have used these products and claim that, in their specific cases, these products are effective in managing their menopause symptoms.

There is limited scientific evidence that many herbs that are listed above actually help menopausal symptoms (see Questions 33 and 36). In fact, many may have potentially harmful side effects and may interact with chemotherapy and other prescribed medications. You always should be cautious when considering herbs because they can have negative health effects. If you are considering using herbal therapy, check with your cancer specialist or clinician. Several Web sites on the Internet discuss herbs, their medical indications and possible interactions, and effects (Memorial Sloan-Kettering Cancer Center, http://www.mskcc. org/aboutherbs; National Center for Complementary and Alternative Medicine, http://www.nccam.nih.com).

Alternative medicine and relaxation techniques can be helpful to minimize hot flashes. Success rates are variable for these techniques to control your symptoms. Their ability to decrease the severity or even prevent hot flashes lacks scientific randomized controlled studies that prove effective. Foot reflexology, magnet therapy, meditation, yoga, and therapeutic massage are all widely used strategies for hot flash relief.

Acupuncture is the ancient Chinese medical system where very thin needles are painlessly and strategically placed into the skin. It is used to help control chronic pain in addition to healing a wide variety of other ailments. Acupuncture works by stimulating specific portions of the nervous system, relieving pain by causing signal transmitters and hormones in the brain to work in different ways. Many women report relief from hot flashes with acupuncture.

Many local and national cancer institutions have excellent integrative medicine departments that specialize in herbal supplements as well as complementary and alternative medicine choices. They can be very helpful in the overall management of your survivorship care. Both Memorial Sloan-Kettering Cancer Center and the M.D. Anderson Cancer Center have excellent resources available in the division of integrative medicine. For more information concerning medical uses of acupuncture, consult the American Academy of Medical Acupuncture on the Internet (http://www.medicalacupuncture.org).

Breathing, focusing on the breath, is as simple a form of meditation as there is, and as effective. Everything I read and hear about meditation says it is good for you. What do you have to lose? I have meditated off and on since college, but I do it regularly now, and without fail. It is a little effort with a big benefit. Wayne Dyer's Getting in the Gap *is a good, easy, and short how-to on meditating, but there are lots of books out there on meditation. Transcendental Meditation is also an excellent and easy method, but there is a cost and formal instruction involved.*

Frances S.

54. Will prescription medications help minimize my hot flashes?

Many medications are available by prescription if you need help with your hot flashes. Talk with your doctor or nurse about your medications to see if you should try another type of medicine and discuss possible side effects. Some prescription medications that can be helpful with troublesome hot flashes include:

- Antihypertensive mediations (clonidine and methyl dopa)
- Antidepressants or the selective serotonin reuptake inhibitors (SSRIs; venlafaxine [Effexor®])
- Paroxetine (Paxil®), an SSRI, has shown success for the treatment of moderate hot flashes. Many women find this medication very helpful in small doses but others who may be very sensitive to this class of drugs may experience negative sexual side effects from SSRI medications.
- Antiepileptics like gabapententin (Neurontin®) also may be an effective pharmacological therapy for the

hot flash sufferer; however, they do have some common side effects. You should avoid alcohol when on this type of medication.

Remember that all medications have some side effects so, in addition to discussing this with your clinician, it is best to carefully read the package insert that comes with the prescription.

55. How can I keep my vulvar and vaginal tissues healthy during my menopause?

In the menopausal transition and as a result of treatment for many cancers, the vulva and the vagina can change in texture. The menopausal period is often accompanied with vaginal dryness and other changes in the perineal area (located between the vaginal opening and the anus in women). The vulva, vagina, and clitoris can become very dry, irritated, and even sore to touch as a result of falling estrogen levels.

To prevent or minimize pain, itching, redness, or burning, skin care of the vulva is important. Menopausal women should be aware that some of these changes can be minimized and that minor changes in perineal and vulvar hygiene can help preserve and prevent further damage to the sensitive area of the female pelvis.

Clothing should minimize vaginal or vulvar irritation. Using a breathable fabric like cotton underwear is the best choice. In the privacy of her own home, some women may prefer not to wear underwear at all. Wear thigh high or knee high hose instead of pantyhose. If you must wear pantyhose, try cutting out the center of the crotch because tight fitting underwear can cause vulvar and clitoral discomfort. Choose loose-fitting pants or skirts, and remember to remove wet bathing suits and exercise clothing promptly.

56. Should I change the way I do my laundry? What about personal and genital hygiene?

The way you clean your undergarments and the way you clean the genitals can definitely influence vaginal health and personal comfort. Some suggestions to help maintain healthy vulvar and vaginal health are listed below.

- Use only mild detergents, such as those that are specifically made for babies, to wash undergarments and underwear. Double-rinse underwear and any other clothing that comes into contact with the vulva. Do not use fabric softener. You want to minimize the amount of harsh chemicals that are left over in any clothing that might irritate the vaginal areas.
- Use soft, white, unscented toilet paper. Pat the vulvar area dry with light pressure only. Do not rub back and forth with pressure; this can create a scratching irritation.
- Some women use lukewarm or cool baths to relieve burning and irritation. Fill your bath with only an inch or two of tepid water. Adding four to five tablespoons of baking soda, colloidal oatmeal (such as Avenal®), or chamomile tea bags to the water may help reduce itching and irritation.
- Abstain from a perfumed bubble bath, feminine hygiene products, or any perfumed creams, sprays,

or soaps. Lotions also should be avoided in the pelvic area.

- Use a soft cloth or your fingers to cleanse the vulva. Wash the vulva with cool to lukewarm water only. If you feel you must use soap, use baby soap or soap for sensitive skin that is mild and unscented. Pat the area dry gently with a soft towel. Again, do not rub.
- Rinse the vulva area completely with water after urination. A small spray bottle filled with cool tap water may make this task easier to do. Urinate often before your bladder is completely full.
- If you are menstruating, be sure to use 100% cotton menstrual pads and tampons. Two brand names that may be helpful include Caracara® and Organic Essentials®, but there may be others on the market as well.

57. Should I change my physical or daily activities to help maintain vaginal health?

The list below contains a few tips that you can follow to help you maintain vaginal health.

- Avoid strenuous exercises that can put direct pressure or tightening on the vulvar tissues such as bicycle riding and horseback riding.
- It may be wise to limit an intense exercise that creates a lot of friction in the vulvar area, especially those that cause the labia major and minor to rub against one another. You may attempt to slow down the intensity of exercises such as walking.
- Use a frozen gel pack wrapped in a towel to relieve symptoms after exercise. Wash and dry the genitals completely after vigorous exercise where you have perspired.

- Enroll in an exercise class such as yoga to learn stretching and relaxation exercises.
- Limit the time you spend swimming in highly chlorinated pools and avoid soaking in hot tubs or very hot baths.
- By drinking plenty of fluids, you will help keep your urine dilute and less likely to sting or irritate the vulvar area.
- Ask your doctor or nurse if it is advisable to use a foam rubber donut if you are engaging in long periods of sitting.
- If you must sit all day at work, try to intersperse periods of standing and exercise throughout the day.

58. My vagina is so dry. How can I keep my vagina tissue healthy?

Starting in the perimenopasual period and progressing into the menopause, the vaginal tissues naturally become dry as a woman's estrogen levels decrease. This can lead to troublesome symptoms of itchiness, burning, irritation, and often leads to painful intercourse. Luckily, there are many methods to treat the symptoms of vaginal dryness or vaginal atrophy.

No estrogens? As women age, the vagina becomes dry and less elastic. Cancer treatments can hasten these changes. Some women can take estrogen either by a pill, patch, cream, ring, or gel to prevent these changes. However, these may not be safe options for many women who have had cancer, especially those with hormonally sensitive cancers. Review the suggestions listed in this section with your doctor or nurse before considering estrogen therapy.

Vaginal moisturizers and lubricants may be helpful in maintaining vaginal health especially for women who decline or are not candidates for hormones. Many products are on the market that may help maintain your vaginal moisture. A simple vitamin E capsule can be punctured with a pin and then inserted into your vagina. (Remember, if you insert the entire capsule into the vagina, the gel cap will come out of the vagina in time.) Another method is to empty the capsule's gel content onto your finger and insert vaginally. Replens® is another vaginal moisturizer that can be purchased over-the-counter and it that comes with an easily filled applicator. You can use either moisturizer two to three times a week. These and other moisturizers are readily available without a prescription in most drug stores or via the Internet. It is important to remember that you may need to wear a panty liner. If you also use a vaginal estrogen product, alternate the days you use a moisturizer. For example, use the moisturizer on Monday, Wednesday, and Friday and the local estrogen product on Tuesday and Thursday. Be sure to read the ingredients of the moisturizers because some can contain bactericides, spermicidal components, colors, flavors, and other additives that can irritate the sensitive vaginal lining. Vaginal moisturizers should be used on a regular basis and are used INDEPENDANTLY of sexual intercourse; they help hydrate the vaginal lining and help restore vaginal elasticity, pliability, and stretchability.

Vaginal lubricants are typically used to make sexual intercourse more pleasurable. Three common examples are Eros® Woman, Astroglide®, and KY® Jelly. A good lubricant should be water-based and compatible with rubber products like diaphragms or condoms. Once applied, they stay moist and sustain lubrication without becoming sticky, goopy, or gummy. They are typically easy to apply within the vagina and often are easy to clean up. Some are goopy while others are slick and slippery. It is best to experiment with different types and determine which you and your partner feel is best during intercourse. Many can be purchased at your local grocery store or over the Internet as well.

Menopausal women with severe **vaginal atrophy** and thinning of the vaginal lining should avoid additives in lubricants like colors, flavors, spermicidal additives, bactericides, or warming ingredients. These can irritate the sensitive vaginal lining. Petroleum-based products such as mineral oil, petroleum jelly, and edible oils or other liquid food products should be generally avoided within the vaginal vault. They can upset the delicate balance between the good and bad bacteria located within the vagina and result in vaginal infections in certain women. These products have also been known to impact the safety and utility of condoms.

What about vaginal hormones? Local vaginal hormones come in a variety of different application methods. Creams, gels, rings, and tablets are the most common types of minimally-absorbed vaginal estrogen products that provide small doses of estrogen directly in the vagina. Vaginal and vulvar creams like Premarin® or Estrace® are typically applied to both the interior of the vagina and exterior of the vulvar vault. Some women find these especially soothing and those with extreme vulvar atrophy and shrinkage may benefit from cream application. Caution should be used with these creams as it is proven that your systemic hormonal levels can increase if using them. The ring (Estring®) is placed within the vaginal vault for three

Vaginal atrophy
when the vaginal tissues decrease in size, become pale or dry without lubrication; this is usually a result of decreased hormones in the woman's body (as in menopause or other medical conditions) which affects these sensitive tissues.

months and then is replaced. This does not work as a pessary (medical device used for pelvic floor defects) and does not help with urinary incontinence (involuntary loss of urine). Some women find this helpful because they do not have to remember to use a product on a daily basis and it is minimally absorbed, but others find it uncomfortable and some partners complain of feeling the ring during intercourse.

Minimally absorbed vaginal tablets (Vagifem®) are another type of vaginal hormone replacement. Vagifem® tablets are contained in a plastic disposable applicator. Insert it into your vagina every night for 14 days. Then insert it twice a week, at bedtime. This medication contains 17 Beta estradiol and comes in convenient prefilled applicators that are biodegradable. A small study in the United Kingdom (only 7 breast cancer patients on both an aromatase inhibitor and Vagifem®) reported increased estradiol levels in the women using Vagifem®. Many women prefer Vagifem® since there is no mess or leakage and it is easy to use. While the study was too small to be valid, and there were several serious flaws with their study, the results are provocative. The long term safety for minimal absorbed vaginal estorgen products needs to be further studied especially in larger populations.

Although many breast cancer patients use minimally-absorbed local estrogen products, their safety in this population appears to be good, but this not been proven scientifically. Whether you actually need a progesterone agent if you are only on a minimally-absorbed vaginal product is controversial. Some health care providers advocate a progesterone agent in women with an intact uterus. Of course, any abnormal vaginal bleeding should always be reported and an immediate comprehensive work up and evaluation should be preformed.

Ask your doctor, nurse practitioner, or other sexual medicine specialists about which type of local estrogen (if any) is appropriate for you.

59. Since my menopause, I sometimes urinate a little when I laugh or cough. How can I strengthen my pelvic floor muscles? What are Kegel exercises?

Leaking urine is a common problem for women as they age. Sometimes women are embarrassed or ashamed about these symptoms, so they fail to mention them to their healthcare professional. However many of the underlying issues can be easily corrected. A small, subclinical urinary tract infection can cause episodic incontinence or loss of urine. Other times, it is because the pelvic muscles need to be strengthened. In this case, there are specific exercises you can do to improve your ability to hold your urine. Remember to urinate often and limit the amount you drink in the evenings if you are waking up to urinate frequently in the middle of the night.

By strengthening your pelvic floor muscles, you can regain control over your loss of urine. These muscles can be identified by voluntarily stopping the stream of urine during mid urination. Another helpful trick is to consciously focus on tightening the muscles you use when you are trying to hold back the expulsion of excessive gas (flatus).

Kegel exercises

exercises designed to increase muscle strength and elasticity in the pelvis; often recommended for the treatment of urinary incontinence.

Kegel exercises are simple to do. During urination, stop the urine in mid stream, hold and count to three or five, and then restart urinating. You should repeat this process several times throughout the day. Try to make a conscious effort not to use your stomach, leg, or buttock muscles because this will not help strengthen your urinary muscles. Your healthcare provider or nurse practitioner can be helpful when you are uncertain if you are contracting the appropriate muscle. These exercises can be done throughout the day, not only when urinating. A total count of 200 per day should be your goal. Tighten the muscles, hold for several seconds then release. Repeat this process. You may do these exercises at any time in the day, and in any position, but many women prefer to do them while lying down or sitting in a chair. You should try to do these exercises for a minimum of six to eight weeks before you notice any improvement.

If you are still having urinary complaints and lose urine during walking, laughing, or straining, you may need a further work up by your gynecologist or urologist. Special medications and testing may be required to help eliminate this troubling condition. Do not delay in seeking therapy and treatment. Most women can be helped with medications, but there are surgical interventions that can prove helpful for the women suffering from severe urinary loss.

PART 7

Mind, Stress, and Time Management

How can I find inner spiritual meaning after cancer?

How can I cope with hair loss and
other physical changes?

What can I do to regain my memory?

What strategies can I use to cope with my stress?

I feel overwhelmed with all that I need to do.
How can I manage my time better?

More ...

Spiritual connectedness for the cancer survivor may take many forms, ranging along the spectrum of a strengthening of faith or resurgence of participation in an organized religion, to a complete and utter loss of faith. Personal belief systems may be at odds, causing the cancer survivor to struggle with their spirituality in the face of their severe and debilitating illness. Others allow their religious beliefs and convictions in a higher being guide them through difficult times.

Surviving a serious illness like cancer is a complex, multidimensional journey that no two women will experience in the same fashion. Patients may question, "why me?" and struggle with why they got cancer in the first place. They often examine past transgressions, wrongs, lies, and/or social behaviors that led them astray and ultimately punished them with cancer. They blame themselves and internalize their anxiety and concern.

When healthcare professionals explain the origin of cancer, discussing the science of proteins, oncogenes, and risk factors, this often does not helps the patient let go of self blame. Often the "why me" question goes unanswered. The ability to accept this unknown is one of the ultimate goals of cancer survivorship.

How can I successfully cope with cancer? Some women embrace survivorship, considering each day as a new and vibrant lease on life. When you were first diagnosed with cancer, it probably overtook your life, and your healing process became a preoccupation that began to dominate your everyday existence. The transition to survivorship is a complex journey. Some fulfill a long list of desires that were once shelved for the tomorrows to come. Many embark on a route of positive thinking and begin Tai Chi, yoga, meditation, and macrobiotic diets. Some believe that bringing holistic mental treatments into the forefront of their survivorship experience is paramount. Others primarily focus on getting back to their normal routine and work schedules as if the illness was just a little blip on their radar, an unplanned glitch or inconvenience along their life's path. The surgery, treatments, and therapies are placed firmly in the past as they reembrace the joys of life and face survivorship in stride. They accentuate the positive in life while minimizing their troublesome experiences.

Yet, many women face survivorship with concern, anxiety, and constant fear. An overwhelming fear of cancer's recurrence can be debilitating. They are stunned and shocked. Some become obsessed with anything that might reduce cancer and have gone as far as eliminating microwaves and televisions in their homes to decrease the amount of radio waves in their environment. These people face cancer survivorship with considerable stress and anxiety, especially on the anniversary of the date of diagnosis or when their treatment was completed.

But survivorship also can bring feelings of new hope, happiness, and even excitement to some women. Living with cancer is a personal journey that each woman experiences in her own way. Give yourself the permission to have a unique journey, a journey of personal growth, learning, and gentle time of healing from your illness experience.

You can ask "why me" all day long and you're not going to get an answer. So you might as well save yourself the trouble and get on with the "now what?" Not to say that you don't get mad as hell and want to throw things. Of course you do. Give yourself some peace and some stillness when you feel angry or frustrated. Breathe. Then get back out there and live. I've always felt like I was here for a reason and that my biggest job in life was to figure out what that was and to do it. Maybe having cancer was part of that for me. I don't like it but I am learning a lot about myself, and about my faith, personal power, compassion, and purpose. Cancer is one heck of a teacher. I figure if something is going to be that much of a pain in the ass, I might as well find some way to benefit from it, and I have.

Frances S.

60. Can complementary medicine play a part in my mental health?

Different types of touch therapies can be incorporated in to your survivorship plan to help keep stress at a minimum and relieve daily tensions.

Reflexology is when pressure is applied in different areas of the foot to relieve stress and pain. Because many of the nerves in the body end in the feet, this technique can promote circulation.

Shiatsu massage involves gentle pressure and slow body stretching to maintain optimum health. *Swedish massage* relieves tension by the masseuse deeply kneading muscles.

Aromatherapy is the ancient art of inhaling specific scents (aromas) to help maintain bodily health. Essential oils are concentrated aromas that can be inhaled to promote a quiet sense of peace. Lavender, rosemary, or

Reflexology

a type of alternative therapy using massage and pressure applied to the foot to relieve stress, pain, and promote circulation.

Shiatsu

a type of massage involving pressure and bodily stretching to maintain optimum health; Swedish massage relieves tension by deeply kneading muscles.

Aromatherapy

the ancient art of inhaling or using specific scents or aromas to help maintain bodily health. Essential oils can be inhaled to promote a quiet sense of peace.

chamomile essence can be purchased at the local store; a few drops in bath water can be especially soothing. Scented candles also may promote a tone of tranquility and peace. Ancient mythology states that when the Pharaoh Cleopatra rode down the Nile river, her boat's sails were soaked in ylang ylang, an aphrodisiac scent, to help lure the Roman general, Mark Anthony. An Austrian study found that the smell of lavender helped some women fall asleep.

Reiki is a type of gentle touch therapy that promotes a sense of calmness and tranquility. This specific touch therapy may help you to reduce anxiety, decrease muscle tension, and maintain an ordered sense of calmness.

Meditation is practiced worldwide among nearly all cultures. Essentially, most styles of meditation involve regulating the breath to still the mind. Many use specific sitting postures, hand positions, or tools (such as a rosary or mala circle of prayer beads; holding a dorje; or repeating a mantra, which is a repeated significant uplifting and/or spiritual phrase) to focus completely on the present. Just as the paced respiration exercise (see Question 51) helped you gain inner calm, meditating can bring serenity to your mind. Using guided imagery during meditation can be helpful also.

Yoga is another popular exercise that many women use to help tone their bodies and relax their minds. Its purpose is to unify the elements of mind and body by doing a series of stretching exercises and holding different postures while deeply breathing. Yoga helps eliminate stress and decrease fatigue.

Music therapy

a therapeutic technique exposing the patient to the pleasures of music, either by listening or playing an instrument, in the company of a psychotherapist specializing in this technique. Creativity, inner peace, and personal pleasure can be enhanced while self-expression can promote an improved sense of well being.

Music therapy is another type of alternative therapy where women can listen to or play a musical instrument in the company of a music therapist. Creativity, inner peace, and personal pleasure can be enhanced while self-expression can promote feelings of well being.

As a professional writer and editor, I'm in the business of creativity. As an amateur painter, avid cook, outdoors-lover, and enthusiast of lots (probably too many) of things, I'm creatively having fun in my after business hours, too. This is not to trivialize all of the serious issues and responsibilities that life with cancer entails, but you don't have to think about them all the time. Doing something that gets you out of your head and into your heart and soul—something that brings you joy—is not just important, but good for you. You hear me? Good for you! It can be a tiny thing: reading a poem, baking a cake, riding a bike. Or a big thing like writing a book. Teaching a class. Climbing Kilimanjaro. I go to the Church of Whatever Works, and anybody can join.

Frances S.

61. I feel sad and am crying a lot. How can I get a handle on my depression?

During your journey through cancer, it is normal to feel low, anxious, or even depressed at different times of your therapy. It is a normal emotion to feel sad and grieve when you believe that you have lost a vital part of yourself and are worried about what the future may hold.

When sadness persists for a long period of time and is combined with feelings of helplessness or hopelessness, and you experience a loss of or increased appetite and sleep disturbances (like insomnia, lack of sleeping, or hypersomnia, sleeping all the time; see Question 47), a diagnosis of major depression may be considered.

When should you seek help for your low moods? The answer is when your emotions interfere with your daily activities. When you are careless of your hygiene, you lack a zest for life, or you withdraw from social and professional commitments, it is time to seek professional help. If you find yourself making plans to hurt yourself or even kill yourself (suicide), seek immediate medical attention.

In our era, depression is not seen as a sign of weakness or stigma. Rather, it is a biological condition. Depression is a medical illness that can be treated effectively with both medications and psychotherapy. Very often, the successful management of depression uses one of many antidepressant medications combined with psychotherapy by a trained **psychiatrist**, psychologist, or social worker.

The cause (etiology) of a major depression is often multifaceted, so it requires a multidimensional approach for truly effective treatment. Biological, psychological, and social factors are often addressed during therapy sessions.

There are many types of therapy. Individual counseling therapy is when you visit with a therapist by yourself; group therapy is when a small number of people meet with a therapist. Cognitive behavioral therapy, interpersonal therapy, supportive psychotherapy, and psychodynamic psychotherapy are different programs that you may consider when talking with your therapist(s).

Psychiatrist
a degreed, credentialed physician who specializes in the prevention, diagnosis, and treatment of mental illness; a psychiatrist can prescribe medicine.

Some women find comfort in talking with other women who have undergone the same treatments or suffer the same type of cancer. Group therapy or a support group is helpful. Many national cancer centers have posttreatment resource centers or survivorship programs that organize group support programs for both men and women, and sometimes they are cancer diagnosis-specific. Other program events can include discussions about depression, sexual health, or other survivorship issues. Sharing your concerns and fears with others may be a way to help you regain control over some emotions that you are experiencing.

62. My appearance has changed and I don't even look or feel like myself. What is the "Look good... Feel better Program®? How can I deal with my new body image?

Changes in appearance are common after cancer and its therapies. If you have had surgery, sometimes your body has new scars. If organs have been removed, often you feel like something is missing. Radiation and chemotherapy can leave you with hair loss or thinning that affects how you feel about yourself (see Question 63).

The Look good... Feel better Program® is a free service provided for women with cancer so that they can learn new ways to restore body image and cope with the changes in appearance that cancer may have caused. This exciting program is a joint venture between the American Cancer Society, the Cosmetic, Toiletry and Fragrance Association Foundation, and the National Cosmetology Association. Certified beauty consultants that are skin, nail care, and hair specialists as well as professional make-up artists educate the cancer survivor about new techniques to enhance her physical image.

Sometimes physical appearance can be linked with self-esteem, so real or imagined body disfigurement may be distressing. Women who have breast cancer surgery may have a different shape and/or altered appearance to their breasts because of the lumpectomy or partial mastectomy. With complete mastectomies (where all of the breast tissue and nipples were surgically removed) and chest wall radiation, the resulting chest may appear disfiguring, which may be disheartening to the female cancer survivor. Surgical reconstruction may not change how a woman feels about her breasts and changed appearance. The survivor may feel ashamed or embarrassed at getting undressed in front of her partner, or even worried about emotional rejection because of her physical changes.

There are many different ways for a woman to regain some sense of femininity while maintaining high fashion. In association with self-esteem exercises and perhaps psychotherapy or psychological counseling, she can choose from an array of special clothing such as bras, lingerie, and sportswear. Sharp looking clothes can help the woman to reclaim a sense of her own special beauty and help her feel attractive.

It is normal for a woman to experience a grief reaction when coming to terms with the fact that she is no longer the same person physically as she was before her cancer diagnosis. She may also grieve that she is no longer able to have more children. The Appendix lists many resources for women coping with body image and regaining self-esteem.

Some women who have ostomies (a bag which is on the outside of the body used to store fecal waste in the event of a colonic or anal resection) are self-conscious concerning the visual appearance of their bag and are concerned regarding foul odors and spillage. These concerns can be distressing and affect how a woman feels about herself and limit her ability to pursue new friendships and sexual relationships. Some suggestions to help women with ostomy concerns include: purchasing new sexy lingerie specifically designed as ostomy covers and changing the bag frequently, especially when anticipating social situations or sexual activity. There are specially designed, odor-controlling tablets that can be placed within the bag to minimize offensive odors. Certain foods that may cause increased odors should be avoided as well. During sexual activity, remember to liberally use pillows and comforters. Choosing sexual positions that are comfortable and place minimal pressure on your ostomy bag is best.

63. I have lost my hair and feel so ugly. How can I cope with my hair loss?

Some women spend many hours brushing, blow-drying, styling, and coloring their hair, so it can be devastating when hair loss is a part of your cancer survivorship. According to the American Academy of Dermatology, by the age of 40 approximately 40% of women have begun to experience some form of hair loss. Hair problems can be on the face (hirsuitism, excessive hair growth), scalp (alopecia, loss of hair), and other areas of the body such as arms and genital area. For some women, hair loss can be thinning all over wheras men may develop a bald spot.

With menopause and lowered estrogen levels or your cancer treatment, you may find yourself with less hair or chronic thinning of your existing hair pattern, especially on the top of the scalp or frontal area. Some women may find benefit from minoxidil (Rogaine®), a topical medication that may stimulate hair follicle growth and increase blood circulation to the scalp, thereby increasing hair growth. Common side effects include itchiness of the scalp, headache, heart palpitations, and mild facial hair growth. Another medical treatment (Propecia®) is an oral prescription medication for hair loss, but is presently not indicated for women with alopecia. An herbal product (Revivogen®) may promote hair growth and prevent further loss or thinning.

Hair transplantation is a surgical procedure that moves hair follicles from one area to another to help lessen thinning. Wigs are another practical suggestion for women who have had hair loss. They are no longer the plastic, fake-looking hair pieces of the past but are very well made and are able to be colored, styled, and personalized to your specifications. Well constructed wigs can be discrete, stylish, and natural looking. You can do most activities without fear of them falling off. Wigs are low maintenance and flexible.

Several nonprofit organizations collect human hair donations so that wigs can be manufactured for cancer survivors. Locks of Love is a well-established nonprofit organization dedicated to gathering donated hair. This group provides hairpieces to financially disadvantaged

Hair transplantation

a surgical procedure that moves hair follicles from one area to another to help lessen thinning hair, particularly on the crown of the head.

children across the United States who suffer from long-term medical hair loss. These children receive custom-made wigs for free or on a sliding scale fee based on need. Wigs for Kids is another nonprofit group that accepts donated hair. This organization also gives hair-pieces to children affected by medical hair loss.

For more information concerning the services that are available in your area or if you would like to enhance your physical appearance, contact the Look better... Feel better Organization on their Web site (http://www.lookbetterfeelbetter.org).

Devastating. Well, yeah, but hair does grow back. And mean-while I do not have to spend hours (and hours) fooling with it to make it look good, or pay somebody to make it look good. I see (and saw) this as a great bonus. It almost made up for the time spent going to doctors' appointments and treatments and radiation and all that. Well, not quite, but almost.

Wigs are great. They really are. The fake-hair ones now are really good. Everyone told me if I got an expensive, custom-made, real-hair wig and an inexpensive fake-hair wig that I would end up wearing the fake one most of the time. I didn't believe it but they were right. Wish I had saved myself the $4,000 or whatever the fancy one cost and just gone with the several-hundred-dollar fake-hair one. There are also in-betweens—wigs that are combinations of real and artificial hair, with varying prices in the hundreds, generally. Check the Internet and Yellow Pages. Go to the wig place and try them on. Have them cut, color, and style it especially for you. That's their job and they like doing it.

Frances S.

64. How can I find inner spiritual meaning after cancer?

The cancer experience can sometimes strengthen a person's faith in a higher being and some people may turn to prayer for spiritual guidance and support. Clergy, ministers, pastors, or rabbis can be wonderful sources of comfort. Those who are ill and their family members may seek out these religious leaders for guidance during troubled times.

Having cancer can be a test of one's religious beliefs and spiritual commitment. Many people seriously question why they got sick, ask why they must suffer from cancer, and face their mortality. Men and women often believe that they need a direction, goal, or a road map of their life that guides their spirituality. Religion can be an enormous support for a spiritual person. Each must journey on their quest for spiritual meaning at her or his own pace.

Some women feel confused, angry, resentful, and/or anxious about their illness. They microfocus in a "Why Me Syndrome" and rave in an endless round of questions such as "why did I get cancer," "why must I be sick now," and "why is my family suffering the consequences of my illness?" Turning guilt and anger inward often leads to depressive symptoms and unhealthy thought processes.

Religion can be a guide for you during difficult times. Think about reconnecting with some form of spiritual meaning. Whether it be talking with your religious leader, an enlightened friend or family member, or experiencing new spiritual pathways, reading religious texts or challenging your faith and belief systems are a few of the healthy ways to explore your inner self. Religion can be comforting and helpful in your spiritual journey of cancer survivorship.

I think if you had "inner spiritual meaning" before cancer, then you will have it afterwards, and maybe even more so. I certainly did. If you didn't have it, the occasion of cancer is a real good time to search for meaning and truth, whatever that might mean to you, if for no other reason than it will make you feel better. Ask around if you think finding "inner spiritual meaning" or a connection to something or someone higher or greater than yourself will help. You'll find somewhere to start; go from there.

Frances S.

65. I have "chemo brain." How can I improve my memory?

With certain chemotherapies, sometimes women complain of increased forgetfulness or loss of memory. If you have experienced this specific problem since your therapy for cancer, there are many things you can do to improve your memory. Certain mental techniques and nutrition may help improve your short- and long-term memory.

Stimulate your memory

Your mind is like any other muscle in your body. You must exercise and use it for it to be strong and healthy. One way to do this is to learn new skills. Teach yourself a new software program on your computer. Take a ballroom dancing class and practice the steps. Go to a home improvement workshop and learn how to tile, fix plumbing, or build a deck. Art classes are fun places to learn how to work clay to throw a pot, paint china, sew, draw, and accomplish a myriad of projects. Play games like chess or backgammon; do crossword puzzles or wonder words. Toy sections of your local stores sell all kinds of card and number (such as the popular **Soduko**) games that you can exercise your number skills alone or play with your family. Picture puzzles are a relaxing way to explore shapes and colors; crossword puzzles help you to recall words and names.

Keep working the brain muscle so it stays fit and healthy. Read new books on a variety of new and exciting topics that interest you. Share a movie or a newspaper article with your partner and then discuss it. Watch a documentary or action adventure movie and try to recall the details of the plot to a friend. The most important issue is to use your memory and help stimulate your brain cells to maintain their health.

Notice everything

Try to focus your attention and concentration on the issues that you believe are most important. Address the details and concentrate. Try to maintain your attentiveness and direct focus. Consciously block out all other distractions.

One fun game is concentration. Place common household objects like a pen, pencil, and safety pin on a tray. Notice their characteristics and texture, their distinct and defining attributes. Try to block out all other distractions as you focus on the objects. Then turn away and recall each one. When meeting new people, notice things about him or her, and then try to associate some detail with their name or personality. For instance,

Sodoku

a type of number puzzle with a 9 × 9 grid subdivided into nine 3 × 3 grids with scattered clues.

Mind, Stress, and Time Management

Mary wears glasses and is a nuclear physicist. Associate her wearing glasses with her highly technical and intricate profession.

Relax and visualize

Attention requires relaxation, so it is imperative that you are relaxed, well rested, and in control of your stress and emotions. Deep, slow, quiet breathing often can help (see the section on paced respiration in Question 51). Take a deep breath in and hold it for 5 to 10 seconds before slowly releasing. Breathe deeply into and out of your diaphragm. Try to see objects in your mind. Use your senses to describe the objects (taste, texture, and touch). Do this with your favorite food. Imagine your favorite restaurant or the smell of your partner's cologne or perfume.

Mnemonics and other memory games

Mnemonics can be very easy ways to remember sequences. A special word is used to remember something, particularly lists. Another technique is alliteration, where the same consonants are repeated in a group of words. Associate a person with an object that rhymes with his or her name. (For example, Michael has black wavy hair that seems to flow in the air when he runs, as if he was riding a motorcycle. Calling him "Motocycle Michael" in your head may help you to remember his name.) Rhyming can help, too. These are very efficient ways to memorize large quantities of information.

Foods, water, and alcohol

A well balanced diet and appropriate nutrition is paramount for an excellently functioning memory. Some believe that certain vitamins may be helpful with memory, most commonly thiamin, folic acid, and vitamin B_{12}. Foods such as bread, cereal, some

Mind, Stress, and Time Management

fruits, and vegetables contain these types of vitamins. Some memory experts believe that vitamins may improve memory, but other healthcare providers have their doubts. No medically sound studies have been preformed to date that document that vitamin supplementation improves either short- or long-term memory.

According to one memory expert, Dr. Carol Trukington, the lack of water in the body has an immediate and deep effect on memory. Dehydration generates confusion and other thought difficulties. Alcohol also can interfere with short-term memory, which will impair one's ability to process and retain new information. Studies show that even drinking small quantities of an alcoholic beverage during one whole week impairs memory. Caffeine in coffee, tea, and chocolate may help you be attentive and end sleepiness; however, excess caffeine results in a state of excitement that interferes with memory function.

Sleep

The brain in particular and the entire human body require time to relax and recover from the stressful day's events. Adequate peaceful and deep sleep is essential for good memory skills. During sleep the mind relaxes, revives, and rejuvenates. Overly stressed or under-rested individuals often complain of having a poor memory. Chronic fatigue, emotional or physical stress, and the lack of complete rest can impair concentration and the ability of the brain to process and retain new information (see Question 47).

Medication

Many medications can contribute to the loss of memory. Some of the common offenders include tranquilizers, muscular relaxants, sleeping pills, and anti-anxiety drugs. The class of drugs that include the benzodiazepines, like diazepam (Valium®) and lorazepan (Ativan®), can contribute to memory problems. Antihypertensive medications that are used to control high blood pressure may not only cause sexual difficulties, but also memory changes and a depressed mood. However, before stopping any type of medication or changing your dosage, it is always advisable to consult your healthcare provider. When stopped abruptly, some medications can cause side effects and symptoms, or even harm you.

Smoking

Smoking cigarettes is a serious health concern. Not only does it contribute to several forms of cancer, particularly in the lungs, mouth, and tongue, but it also decreases the amount of oxygen delivered to the brain. This is another reason to quit smoking now!

66. What practical techniques can I use to help with my memory?

There are many creative memory aids that you can use to remember important names, places, stories, and words used in your daily living. Each time you use any one strategy on the list below, you are creating or strengthening neural pathways in your brain that will help you learn and remember more easily.

1. *Write.* Writing something down takes it out of your mind and makes it a paper or computer record that can be easily remembered. Make notes as someone is saying something you want to remember. Write down and review lists. Keep a personal journal of important things you want to remember and/or events that occur.

2. *Organize.* Sort your papers and throw away what you no longer need. Have baskets, labeled file folders in filing cabinets, or another type of organizing system to sort papers like bills, instruction manuals, and papers that you want to keep. Decluttering your home and office helps calm your mind. Most people feel quite satisfied after their space has been cleaned and organized.

3. *Schedule.* Keep a calendar and write down your appointments and things you regularly do each month. It is much easier to review what you will do each day when your activities are written out. When new things come up, it is easier to cluster activities or make decisions about whether you are able to do them now or later, or not at all.

4. *Notepads.* Place many notepads (each with a pen or pencil) around your home and/or office. When you want to remember something, grab your notepad and jot it down. Later, whatever you wrote can be added to your calendar or tucked into its appropriate file at your convenience.

5. *Memory strategies.* Use memory aiding techniques (see Question 65).

6. *Shopping List.* Before you go shopping, list the items you want to purchase to avoid having to remember too many things.

67. These techniques are not working. Where can I get help?

If you have tried all of these techniques and still have some serious concerns about your recent loss of memory, then it is time to consult a memory specialist for some specific tests. Disorders in memory can interrupt your quality of life. If your memory loss is severe and troubling, perhaps it is caused by a more serious underlying medical issue. Menopause, hormonal or vitamin deficiencies, mental depression, infections, and dementias all can affect mental function and memory. There are many memory and aging facilities that specialize in assessment, diagnosis, and treatment of memory disorders. Ask your primary care physician if a referral is right for you.

STRESS AND TIME MANAGEMENT

68. Why am I so stressed out?

Even though men would like to believe that they are enlightened people of the twenty-first century, clearly, the vast majority of childrearing, cooking, cleaning, and household management still falls on the shoulders of women. This household care, combined with professional responsibilities of work, and extended family as well as child care may tax the already overwhelmed woman. It is no wonder that many women feel as if there is not enough time in the day.

Life stressors tend to build up over time. Often anxiety can spiral out of control. With the advent of portable laptops, computers, Blackberries, and cell phones, we are now jamming more everyday tasks into one 24-hour period. Women tend not to rest. We do not enjoy leisure time because we are preoccupied with all of the details involved in creating fun activities for the rest of our family, or responding to crises, or are thinking about and preparing for the next busy day. We have forgotten to set limits of work and play. Office and home have become blurred.

Stress often feels like you are climbing up a spiral staircase that leads to nowhere. Unfortunately, stress can lead to serious health problems like exhaustion, fatigue, depression, and insomnia.

69. How can I manage my stress better?

Managing stress is a skill that can be learned. While much stress is out of your control, how you organize yourself to respond to stress will directly relate to your quality of life. The following are suggestions of how you can manage your time and thought processes.

Revise your thinking.   When you feel you are at the end of your rope, acknowledge it. Accept the things you can not change. Forgive. Stop and consider if there might be more positive solutions to the problem. When you feel frustrated or tired, take a break. It does not have to be long, but doing so will help you return to the problem with more clarity. Sometimes the solution is staring you in the face. All you need is a short cooling off period to help you discover the best course of action.

Choose a healthy diet and exercise regimen.   Following a diet rich in fruits, grains, and vegetables while decreasing saturated fats tends to lower your blood pressure (see Questions 32–36). Limit caffeinated drinks because they can increase anxiety and cause rapid heart rates. Choose healthy, low calorie snack foods (not fatty foods with empty calories). Your energy and zip will return after eating a nutritious diet. Exercise away your stress (see Questions 37–41). Often a brisk walk or a session at the gym will help clear your mind to the point where you can reframe your problems more creatively and manageably.

Plan. It is always important to stay focused and organized in the face of an action packed day of chores and responsibilities. If you plan your day in advance, you are more likely to spend your time efficiently. Be sure to leave work at your designated time, delegate chores to family members (including children), or (if financially possible) hire extra housecleaning help. Your spouse or partner can always pitch in to get the dry cleaning, shop for food, or help the children do their home wok. Divide and conquer household tasks.

Set limits. Ask yourself, it is really crucial that your bed be made every single day? Is it OK to have some clothes on the floor once in a while? Choose not to get overly stressed if your home is not clean. Make active decisions to delay certain chores.

Say no. Overextending yourself leads to increased stress and anxiety. Learning to say no, at appropriate times, to personal, social, or employment commitments is crucial. Be polite, yet firm in your convictions, to not overextend your schedule. By saying no to certain projects, you remain focused on the activities that are most important to you now.

Relaxation Techniques. Meditation, yoga, or other relaxation techniques provides you with a useful tool to help maintain an active lifestyle with a sense of tranquility, relatively free of stress (see Question 60). Stretching and Tai Chi classes are often offered inexpensively at your neighborhood YMCA or recreation center. Practicing deep breathing for five to ten minutes at a time can be helpful. Lie down on your back in a quiet dark place, take a deep breath in from your diaphragm, hold it for ten seconds, and then release. During this time, try to clear your mind of all thoughts and concerns, and just focus on your breath. Relax your muscles as you inhale and exhale, while letting your mind go completely blank. This exercise is a great stress buster early in the morning or late at night.

There are many other therapeutic strategies available. Professional counseling with a trained social worker, psychologist, or psychiatrist may help you work through childhood issues affecting your life now. Emotional patterns and responses to serious life events can emerge from the subconscious to the fully conscious adult in a safe way for healing. Getting a perspective from a professional therapist often opens new avenues of thinking about your situation. They specialize in helping you develop coping strategies tailored to meet your emotional needs. Question 70 offers additional types of therapies that may be available in your area.

70. What is laughter therapy? How can it help my survivorship journey?

Although cancer is not a laughing matter, **laughter therapy** involves facing adversity with humor. Through humor, you can attack and embrace your cancer experience, and perhaps find a new path on life's journey.

Tania Katan's book, *My One Night Stand with Cancer* is a humorous look at the devastating experience of losing a breast to cancer. Advocates believe that laughter therapy helps you gain physical and mental benefits from laughter. These include lowered blood pressure, decreased anxiety and stress hormones, release of

Laughter therapy

a type of treatment based in the premise that the patient gains physical and mental benefits from laughter, including lowered blood pressure, decreased anxiety and stress hormones, release of endorphins (the body's natural pain killers), and a general sense of well-being.

endorphins (the body's natural pain killers), and a general sense of well being. Some researchers have found that laughter can actually help strengthen your immune response by increasing the number of infection-fighting cells, which helps your body's ability to fight off and even prevent disease.

Laughter therapy formally originated in North America in the 1970s when Norman Cousins recovered from a serious illness (ankylosing spondylitis) after watching comedy shows like "The Marx Brothers" and "Candid Camera." According to his book, *Anatomy of an Illness*, ten minutes of hearty laughter gave him at least two hours of pain relief. In the 1930s, clowns were brought into the children's hospitals to entertain and amuse young people who were afflicted with polio. A 1998 film starring Robin Williams, where humor was used as therapy, was based on the real Hunter "Patch" Adams. Adams is the founder of the "Gesundheit! Institute," the mission of which is to bring fun, friendship, and joy back into healthcare service.

Memorial Sloan-Kettering Cancer Center and many other national and international cancer centers have developed Circus Clown Care Programs for pediatric oncology patients. These programs combine circus artistry, music, and magic tricks with the healing power of humor. So-called "Doctors of Laughology" use comedy, practical jokes, silly instruments like kazoos, music, and magic to help young patients and their families through the difficult journey of cancer care. Laughter can often be the best medicine during and after cancer care. Tell a funny joke or watch a funny movie. Laugh out loud as if no one is watching!

71. Are other types of therapy helpful?

Most cancer centers have access to a broad network of services and staff who can help you tap into resources in your locality. Exploring new strategies outside of your routine can be fun as well as therapeutic.

Art therapy. The creative process of physically making an art project often helps to relieve stress as well as access deep-seated feelings in a safe expression. This is based on the concept that art encourages self-expression, which may help you resolve internal conflicts,and develop better interpersonal skills and communication. Drawing, painting, sculpture, photography, and other art forms are used in association with counseling. Playing in different art mediums is a great way to relax and unwind and will provide many hours of fun. If you are not interested in formalized art therapy, think about reexploring your interest in the arts. Visit a museum, take in a concert, or grab your camera and take photographs. Exploring and reconnecting with art that is all around you can provide you with enormous enjoyment as well as the pleasure of self-expression

Art therapists are specially trained professionals who facilitate art therapeutically; most have a masters degree or higher. This means that they have fulfilled specific educational requirements that include counseling. For more information about how art therapy can help your journey of cancer survivorship, contact the American Art Therapy Association (Web site, http://www.arttherapy.org).

Pet therapy. Enjoying time and leisure activities with your pet is one way to improve your general health through **pet therapy**. Whether it is a dog, cat, parakeet,

Pet therapy

a therapeutic strategy that helps a patient get involved with a dog, cat, or other type of pet; enjoying time and leisure activities with the pet helps the patient's general health.

gerbil, or other, pets can be a soothing addition to any household. Your pet can provide hours of entertainment as well as offer companionship and unconditional love and attention.

Music therapy. Classical music can be soothing and help relax your mind. Some healthcare professionals advocate classical music as a mild sedative. A few composers who wrote serene classical music include Bach, Beethoven, Mozart, and Schubert. Sample New Age, Native American, and World Music sections of the music department in your local store or on the Internet to choose more contemporary soothing tapes and CDs. Some people enjoy the sounds of rain, jungle noises, or birds chirping. Music should be an active part of your everyday life. Listen and relax.

72. What is time management and how can I manage my time more effectively?

Deadlines, schedules, social and personal commitments combined with business obligations, and other family responsibilities can make even the most organized person feel overwhelmed. Over-scheduling adds unnecessary stress to your already hectic life, which can make you feel overwhelmed, anxious, or even depressed (see Question 68).

The essence of time management involves setting limits and prioritizing responsibilities. This may mean that you need to look at the global picture. You must recognize that you cannot continue to say yes to everyone. You cannot be everything to everyone at all times.

To understand and manage your time more effectively, the first thing to do is to write out a personal time survey. This is a list of what you do each day and how long it takes to do it. Look at the time spent sleeping, eating, grooming, commuting to and from work, socializing, child care, etc. Next, set up a daily and then a weekly calendar. How do you spend your day? Can you consolidate activities to minimize travel? Are there errands you can do because they are close to each other? For example, go to the dry cleaners before food shopping because they are located so close together. Can you shop for groceries once a week instead of every day?

Consider consolidating, delegating, or eliminating activities that zap your energy and/or take too much time. It may be necessary to cut down on your personal and professional commitments. Take the time to examine what is important in your life. Those are the activities to fit into your day.

Understanding that your "in box" will always be filled is another key issue. Most people believe that if they only had three to five more hours per day, they could spend more quality time with their children and spouse, not feel so rushed, or keep the house tidier. Clearly knowing your personal priorities is crucial so you can make time to accomplish those goals. You probably will need to simplify your life. Facing the situations of having an hour to finish some work from your business or going to your daughter's ballet practice or son's softball game can be agonizing. Making informed, intelligent choices and understanding that all choices have repercussions that impact your future happiness will help you realize that life is a series of choices. You can make the best decisions for yourself and negotiate choices with your family and all those in your sphere of influence.

Time saving tips

Learn to say no. Too many social and professional responsibilities is overwhelming. Your willingness to say no will help you pick those activities that fit your schedule and interests (see Question 69).

Do not be a perfectionist. Perfection is impossible. Once you release yourself from the inner demand that you must be perfect, you will be much happier coping with reality. Set challenging, attainable goals, relax, and forgive yourself for not being perfect.

Prioritize. What is important to you? Listing and then analyzing all the activities you wish to accomplish will help you place them in the order of importance. What is more important: doing the laundry, visiting with friends, doing a family project, or completing an errand? Only you can reconcile the choice or be flexible depending on the circumstances of your day. Make a "to do list" and follow your daily or weekly planner. Write down your appointments, meetings, and other obligations in an organized manner and try not to deviate from your preset timetable. A fifteen minute visit with your Grandma is a fifteen minute visit. Do not allow it to develop into a two-hour gossip session.

Combine activities. Set a list of activities that need to be completed within a time frame and see if they can be grouped together. Combining activities can help you stay organized and also save time.

Eliminate activities. It is best to eliminate activities that are not productive and often drain your energy. Doing activities begrudgingly or with a bad attitude wastes your time and makes you unproductive.

Delegate. It is important to allow yourself permission to ask others for help. Asking your spouse or partner and other family members to do specific chores, run errands, or support you with child care helps you manage your time more effectively. If you are able to hire someone to help with house and yard work, your time will be freed to do other, more enjoyable things.

Mind, Stress, and Time Management

PART 8

Relationships

How can I help my family? My caregivers?
My loved ones?

Can cancer and the workplace mix?

What about dating and safer sex for
the single cancer survivor?

More...

73. So much has happened. Help me to identify my feelings after cancer.

Social interactions change once you have cancer and its associated therapy. Many experience increased difficulty in the workplace or at school and find it awkward to interact with their colleagues and friends. Cancer can be a time of isolation and loneliness.

You may have workload limitations and may get tired before completing your assigned tasks. Others face job loss, promotion denials, or even discrimination. There is no right or wrong way to feel after your experience with cancer. Many need time to gain knowledge of how to cope with this life-threatening situation.

Women cope with their disease in many different ways. Some actively seek out information and become proactive in their healing process while others simply accept their illness and do not question the therapies. Some maintain an optimistic and realistic vision of themselves and their prognosis. While some find social network support groups such as peer-based social support, others use individual psychotherapy to help them cope.

Every cancer journey is unique. You cannot rush how you are feeling. Take time to explore your feelings. Keeping a journal or setting up a video diary can help record your thoughts and feelings and can be reviewed later. Enjoy your journey of self-exploration.

I don't suppose you ever feel quite the same after having cancer. Even if the doctors say they've "gotten it all," the fact of it lingers. You know it happened, and you know it can happen again. Not a great thing to have hanging over your head. And hanging. But you don't have to stand there under it all the time, either, now do you?

What I don't always know is how other people feel about me after having cancer. Do they see me as weak? Sickly? As "damaged goods"? Some probably do. I can't remember who said, "What other people think of me is none of my business," but it's a great saying. And the truth is that other people are not sitting around thinking about me all that much anyway. They might gossip about me for a few minutes, but then they'll go right back to thinking about themselves and their own problems, like they always do.

As a practical matter, I didn't tell the people I worked with about having cancer. I am a self-employed freelance writer, and I didn't want editors to avoid giving me assignments because they didn't think I was up to it. I wanted to make that decision, thank you. So I kept word of my health status to close friends and family. Now you can't always control what people know about you, but I let it be known that I wanted to be very low key about it. As I said earlier (see Question 4), I didn't want it to be what my life was about. I also didn't want to exhaust myself talking about it to people I wasn't close to.

Another thing that changes after cancer is how you feel about other people, namely friends and family who may— or may not—have been a great support to you. Cancer is nothing if not a test of character, for the patient and for the patient's family and friends as well. Yes, some people will perceive you differently, or even fearfully, because you've had cancer. And while it is well and good to say they feel this way because of their own fears and insecurities, I think it is also due to a lack of character. I wouldn't necessarily end a relationship over it, but I would see it differently and value it less, frankly.

Frances S.

74. How can I help my family? My caregivers? My friends and loved ones?

Cancer affects not only the patient, but also family, friends, coworkers, and acquaintances. If a family member who has cancer is returning home, the emotional dynamics of the household may have changed. The cancer survivor's partner may experience anger, fear, frustration, and even depression or feelings of helplessness.

Sometimes silence is the only way a person can cope. Do not feel badly if someone asks you about your cancer and you do not feel up to chatting or discussing how you are feeling. Politely explain that now is not the best time for you, and you would prefer not talking about it right at this very moment. Remember to always express your appreciation that others are interested in your well being. Most people mean well, but they have a difficult time expressing themselves.

Open communication is the best way to cope with your significant relationships and move forward from the cancer experience in tandem with your husband, boyfriend, or lover. Practically speaking, this translates to doing normal tasks together such as cooking, housecleaning, actively participating in child care, and attending doctor's visits together.

Partners need to spend time just with each other. Honest talking and silent listening (listening to another without interruption) provides an emotional presence and serves as poignant support for the female cancer survivor. Empathy is when your partner sincerely tries to experience your thoughts and feelings without judgment or rash conclusions. Sometimes the best support a partner can provide is allowing the woman to be herself and not try to "fix" her. Whether she is angry, sad, or crying hysterically, a partner's ability to be silent and listen if that is what she needs, lets her know that you will be there for her no matter what.

Communication can break down between partners when one is facing a serious medical disease. Some important ways to enhance communication include taking a walk together, spending time watching TV, reading side-by-side, or just being in each other's company. Ask questions and do not be afraid to hear the answers. Use the word *cancer*. Enjoy silence together. Nonverbal communication like hugging, kissing, and a gentle touch often conveys deeper thoughts and emotions than words.

Relationships and friendships may change drastically once you have been diagnosed with cancer. Friends who were once very supportive and active participants in your life may now choose to be silent and limit their interaction with you. Your cancer diagnosis may stimulate some of their internal fears about death and serious illness, or may even evoke some unpleasant emotions about their own personal experiences with cancer or disease. It is always best to acknowledge your feelings of abandonment and talk with your supportive friends if the time is available. Embrace your feelings of hurt and loss of a close friend and try to understand their position rather than condemn their actions.

Some people may not know how to interact with you. They feel uncomfortable with your new appearance or may not know how calm you are in discussing your cancer. Sometimes insincere, trite, or cruel comments are hurtful. Focus on the fact that in their own way they are attempting to interact with you. A few individuals who have cancer often tell of the story that other people come up to them and say that he or she "has gotten cancer to become a better person," or to realize that there is a lot of positive in the world. Rather than condemn these individuals or become angry with them, realize that often people who are close to you and care for your feelings are at a loss for words. They are too shocked or even horrified with the notion of your illness, and, on some level need to rationalize your sufferings.

Cancer is beyond understanding for many people. Often their comments are rationalizations for their own peace of mind and do not have anything to do with you or your actions. Many people cannot comprehend the issues of why cancer affects certain people. Unfortunately, the mean neighbor down the street may win the lottery and good people get cancer and suffer. It is best to simply embrace your inability to understand things in life. Accept the concept that cancer just happens, it is a disease without discrimination, and it is not a punishment for some past transgression or bad deeds.

It is important to know that there are supportive environments for caregivers and extended families, including children of all ages, and they can access these groups to help with the survivorship journey of their loved one. These groups talk about the difficult discussions that mothers must have with their children about their illness. They help women explain why mother is ill and sometimes cannot play with them. Supportive counselors and therapists can help children through their mother's journey through survivorship. There are also many children's books and audiovisual materials that can help parents explain the illness of cancer to children and other family members.

75. How can partners get a break from cancer?

Just like the patient who has had the disease, spouses and partners of those who had cancer often suffer from many conflicting emotions. They may feel angry, depressed, and saddened by the entire process the illness has taken on the family. Partners may also believe that they need to be the strong, solid one for their loved one and family. Somehow, their emotions are not as important. This need to hide or bury their emotions is often combined with feelings of help-lessness because they feel powerless to completely eliminate the cancer. They must present a brave front and not show signs of depression or worry. Your can-cer center may provide peer support groups for fam-ily members to express their feelings in a nurturing environment.

Often partners of cancer survivors need a "vacation" from cancer. Some coping strategies are reading, hob-bies, listening to music, exercising, movies, and spend-ing time with family and friends. Organized religious events and gatherings also may be a nice and wel-comed outlet.

76. Can cancer and the workplace mix?

Your coworkers may react differently to your having cancer. Some choose to avoid the situation and not mention your illness; they may act as if your absence from work was routine and had no significance or importance. Others may want to discuss your illness with you but are uncertain how you may react to their questions. If your career was important to you before your cancer diagnosis, then returning to work may be an important facet of your survivorship. You may need to work again to reclaim your sense of purpose and help boost your feelings of self worth.

Returning to work may provide you with the needed stability and predictability you lacked when you were ill and in treatment. Although you may feel back to normal and fully recovered, your coworkers may still feel tender or uneasy around you. They may not know how to react or what to say. Accept this behavior and when the appropriate opportunity arises, try to talk to your colleagues concerning their feelings.

If for some reason your cancer and its therapy have left you unable to return to your previous job, then perhaps it is the opportunity to be retrained in another completely different field that sparks your interest. If you always wanted to be involved in the art field then perhaps now is the time to seek out employment in an art gallery. If finances permit, then perhaps it is the best time not to return to work but rather to commit to furthering your education or training. Although it may be stressful to seek new employment, you should look at it as a new exciting adventure where there are endless innovative possibilities and opportunities for exploration.

If health insurance and possibilities of future job availability are an issue, it is best to consult with your healthcare provider. The American's Disability Act protects cancer survivors from job or employment discrimination. Because laws vary from state to state or county to county, it is always advisable to consult your attorney or your local government agency. The American Cancer Society can be an invaluable asset for helping survivors in the workplace. Web sites, organizations, and foundations can be accessed that can provide practical guidance and assistance.

If you do decide to reveal your condition to your coworkers, or if doing so is unavoidable, I think the best defense is a good offense. Meet it head-on. Talk to your coworkers and tell them what you and they can honestly expect. But keep it short and matter-of-fact. Tell them it doesn't change your personality or who you are, and you hope they'll have enough respect and maturity to treat you like they understand that and not to look at you as if you've suddenly sprouted another head. Tell them how much you appreciate their support. Say something funny and self-deprecating. It will lighten the mood. Nervous laughter is better than no laughter at all.

Frances S.

77. What about dating and safer sex for the single cancer survivor?

Women and men are now living longer and have stronger active lives and so are demanding an improved quality of life. Just as before their illness, cancer survivors want to have productive and healthy relationships with a member of the opposite sex or same sex (if they are lesbian), and they want intimate and emotional connections. By thinking and acting in a positive fashion, you will project the image that you want a complete healthy lifestyle that includes a mate or partner. Others will sense your commitment to living an active healthy life and wanting to be a part of it. You should not be denied a mate or love interest just because you have had cancer. If you desire an intimate sexual connection with another person, then you should actively seek this type of human connectedness.

One of the difficult issues that single women face is about disclosure. When is it appropriate to discuss your illness with a potential partner? When should you mention that you only have one breast and will look different if naked? When should you discuss your possible infertility or decreased longevity? There is no right or wrong time to discuss these issues; it depends on the woman and her level of comfort with this new partner. It is important to understand that not all potential partners will be supportive and accept that you have cancer. Those who are emotionally unable to handle your illness will reject you and end the relationship. Know that this is not your issue but rather their insecurity.

With more and more women entering the dating scene after cancer and the prevalence of sexually transmitted diseases (STDs), there is a great concern about safer sex practices. It is always important to communicate with your partner and discuss the issues of birth control and STDs.

Hormonal contraception may not be an option for you because of hormonally sensitive tumors or cancer, so the best choice may be using barrier contraception or condoms. Condoms come in all shapes, sizes, colors, and even flavors. Spermicides or lubricant can be added as well along with ribbing to enhance female pleasure during intercourse. Synthetic latex-free condoms are available for those who are latex-sensitive (Durex Avanti®, Trojan Supra®, eZon®, and Tactylon®). Most brands of condoms are available at your local pharmacy, supermarket, or on the Internet for the discrete shopper.

Sexuality is discussed in more depth in Questions 87–100.

Ooooh boy. A groovy single chick with an active social life in New York City. With breast cancer. Which is very not groovy. I just decided I would hold my head high, wig and all, and keep myself out there in the dating world as much as I felt up to it. I usually waited until I'd gotten to know him a bit to talk about the cancer. And if it never got that far, then it wasn't an issue anyway. If he ended the relationship because he was put off by the cancer, then I don't want that kind of person in my life anyway, to tell you the truth. And to be perfectly honest, I do believe this happened a couple of times (and one of them was a doctor!). But listen, this is the kind of thing I want to know about someone sooner rather than later. Anyone can be a fair weather friend. I want the through-thick-and-thin kind of friend, and so do you.

Right now I'm in a relationship. Now the question becomes what if we stay together, or marry, and the cancer comes back? We have to talk about this. He could be in the position of becoming my caretaker. It's a big deal. It's also worth pointing out that he might get cancer, or be hit by a

bus, or God knows what, and that I might become his care-
taker. They don't put that line in there about "in sickness or
in health" for nothing. I'm not a therapist, but it seems to
me you need to figure this out about anyone you are seri-
ously involved with. And if you don't like what you've fig-
ured out, then bye-bye birdie.

If you're single, first you worry about the dating, and then
you worry about the sex. I was seriously worried about los-
ing my sex drive and/or my sex appeal. The damn cancer's
bad enough, and I've got to lose my "mojo" too?! Please. I
was totally unprepared for this, and my doctors didn't
bring it up until I asked. Perhaps they understandably
didn't want to burden a patient with more not-so-great
news than she was already dealing with. Perhaps this is
less an issue for some than for others, but it was a big one
for me. For example, a common symptom of menopause
(resulting from chemo, in my case) is vaginal dryness,
which can cause pain during intercourse. After several
months' abstinence, I became sexually active again about
halfway through the four-month chemo treatment.
OUCH! I had no idea the vagina would not only be drier
but would lose some of its elasticity. The good news is that
it doesn't have to be or stay that way. Apart from using
lubricants, you can use vaginal dilators and good old-fash-
ioned dildos and vibrators to keep yourself in sexual shape.
(The Internet is full of sources for these things—it's a riot!)
I was mortified to broach the sexuality subject with a doc-
tor, but I was even more mortified at the prospect of a
crummy sex life and refused to accept it. "Use it or lose it,"
my doctor said, "and keep those 'neural pathways' open and
flowing." In other words, keep having orgasms, self-
induced or otherwise. Now that's my kind of prescription.

If your doctor is less than enthusiastic about discussing this
and not offering practical (if embarrassing) advice, then

ask to be referred to someone who is. The specialists—be they physicians, therapists, or counselors—tend to talk about sex very matter-of-factly, like it was the laundry or something, and it makes you able to discuss it matter-of-factly also. (Almost.)

P.S. And if anyone's asking, yes, I definitely kept my wig or scarf or whatever on during The Act, lest I burst into my "Kojak" impersonation at just the wrong moment. You have to be careful about swinging from the chandelier and stuff like that, but otherwise, those wigs stay on pretty well.

Frances S.

PART 9

Fertility

Is pregnancy safe after cancer?

What are the options to preserve my fertility?

Are there other options for me to become a parent?

What other fertility considerations should
I think about?

More ...

I am grateful to the organization, Fertile Hope, which was instrumental in writing this section of the book. They have a plethora of written materials and pamphlets which are an excellent source of information and can be helpful in understanding fertility concerns for the cancer patient. Fertile Hope was founded by a two-time, young adult cancer survivor. Fertile Hope is a national nonprofit organization dedicated to providing reproductive information, support, and hope to cancer patients and survivors. Through programs of awareness, education, financial assistance, research, and support, Fertile Hope is helping cancer survivors fulfill their parenthood dreams.

78. Where do I begin?

If you have been recently diagnosed with cancer, you should know that cancer treatment may affect your fertility, which is your ability to have children. Your oncologist or oncology nurse should explain how fertility may be affected by cancer treatment and your options for being a parent. By understanding your options, you will be able to make informed decisions.

Oncologist

a degreed, certified physician who specializes in treating cancer. Surgical oncologists specialize in cancer surgery; medical oncologists specialize in treatment with chemotherapy, hormonal therapy, and biological therapy; radiation oncologists specialize in treatments with radiation.

Cancer treatments have changed a lot over the last few years. More people with cancer are surviving than ever before. What this means is that many men and women with cancer can look forward to improved quality of life and being a parent after cancer. New treatments may increase your chances of having children. An honest discussion with your healthcare team not only will help you plan your cancer treatment but anticipate possible fertility problems. A few of the health professionals that should be able to help you include your **oncologist**, surgeon, OB/GYN, and a reproductive endocrinologist. Consult your insurance company about the coverage offered for fertility-preserving methods.

Of course, you may feel overwhelmed by all the important decisions you have to make. Not only are you dealing with a new cancer diagnosis and planning your treatment, but you also are thinking about your future fertility. This can be a very stressful and anxious time. Social workers, support groups, and religious advisors can often offer support, guidance, and comfort.

79. What is infertility?

Infertility is not being able to begin (conceive) or complete a pregnancy for the nine months. In more simple terms, a woman is no longer able to become pregnant because her ovaries are no longer producing reproductive hormones (like estrogen and progesterone) or her uterus is unable to hold or maintain the fetus for the duration of pregnancy. Women can be considered infertile when their ovaries cannot produce mature eggs or when damage to their reproductive system prevents an egg from being fertilized or from growing inside the uterus.

Infertility can be temporary or it can last for the remainder of a woman's life. For example, a person receiving chemotherapy may be infertile during treatment but become fertile again after her treatment is completed. Infertility can affect both men and women. In order to better understand how cancer and its treatment can affect fertility, it is helpful to know something about the reproductive system for women.

Female reproductive organs include the uterus (womb), cervix (the opening to the womb at the top of

Endocrinologist
a degreed, certified physician who specializes in diagnosing and treating hormone disorders.

Fertility

Infertility
an inability to begin (conceive) or complete a pregnancy for the entire nine months (gestation). In more simple terms, a woman is no longer able to become pregnant because her ovaries are no longer producing reproductive hormones like estrogen or progesterone that can mature an egg, or her uterus is unable to hold or maintain the fetus for the duration of a pregnancy.

the vagina), fallopian tubes, and ovaries (organs that make eggs and hormones). The female hormones that are involved in the menstrual cycle include estrogen and progesterone. These hormones are help the ovaries and eggs mature, and they are involved in the cyclical development of monthly menstrual periods. During a woman's reproductive years, a woman's ovaries produce eggs that travel in the fallopian tubes to the uterus. If the mature egg is fertilized by a male sperm and implants within the uterus, a pregnancy can result. If implantation does not occur, the endometrial lining of the uterus deteriorates and the lining flows out of the body as menstruation.

80. Should I have children after my cancer? Is pregnancy safe after cancer?

According to the American Cancer Society's new information booklet, *Fertility and the Cancer Patient*, some doctors think that pregnancy after cancer can be safe but other doctors do not agree. Because every cancer is different, it is difficult to make a broad statement that pregnancy is safe for all cancer survivors. If you are thinking about becoming pregnant after cancer, discuss your plans with your healthcare team. Your doctor can talk with you about your personal health risk, chance of tumor recurrence, and the impact that pregnancy and parenthood may have on your cancer care.

After receiving a cancer diagnosis, many wonder if they should even consider having children. Many women who have cancer question whether there is a genetic factor that caused them to get cancer and if they will pass on this "cancer gene" to their children. Concerns about the cancer returning and the health and financial burdens of raising a child along with medical and healthcare concerns are some of the critical issues that cancer survivors face when thinking about having children.

Underlying mental illness like complaints of depression, anxiety, and stress may limit a person's capacity to make a well thought out decision about her reproductive choices. These serious questions should be discussed with those you feel comfortable with: your spouse or partner, healthcare team including your oncologist and surgeon, mental healthcare professional, family, and even close friends or religious leader. There are also many support groups as well as health professionals (see the Appendix) who focus on reproductive and fertility issues with the person with cancer.

81. How does cancer treatment affect my fertility?

Some, but certainly not all, cancer treatments affect your ability to have children. The effect of treatment on fertility depends on the type of cancer you have, the stage of diagnosis, and the associated treatment you receive. Of course, different people respond to different therapies differently. Some personal characteristics, like your age and general health, are also very important.

Chemotherapy and fertility. Chemotherapy is the use of medications (drugs) that target and destroy rapidly dividing cells throughout the body, including human cells that are not affected by cancer. Healthy cells in the reproductive organs can be damaged by the chemotherapy treatments. In men, chemotherapy damages the testicles and may kill sperm or reduce their ability to move. In women, chemotherapy may damage the ovaries and eggs. This damage can result in a disease called *premature ovarian failure* (when the ovaries cannot produce hormones or mature eggs) and menopausal symptoms like hot flashes and vaginal dryness. According to the American Cancer Society's Fertility and the Cancer Patient booklet, women who have cancer during their childbearing years have between a 40% and 80% chance of becoming infertile. Women whose cancer was treated before age 30 often have the best chance of becoming pregnant after completion of chemotherapy; however, the woman or young teenage girl who goes into premature menopause because of chemotherapy may not be able to get pregnant.

The type of chemotherapy, dosage, frequency of treatment, and age may all contribute to the type and severity of damage that is done to your eggs. If your doctor has recommended chemotherapy as your treatment, ask if your chemotherapy will affect your egg quality or quantity. The encouraging news is that some women who seem to be infertile during treatment or immediately after therapy may improve and become fertile again after their chemotherapy is completed. At a minimum, women are typically advised not to get pregnant within the first year after receiving chemotherapy because the medicine may have damaged their eggs. According to some research, this could result in miscarriage or genetic problems with their babies. This damage seems to be repaired after about six months. Other physicians advocate waiting a longer period before attempting to get pregnant. Discuss your unique situation with your oncologist and your heathcare team.

Radiation therapy and fertility. Radiation therapy uses high-energy particles to destroy or damage a cancer cell; pelvic radiation can affect the ovaries, eggs, or follicles. Only the tumor and surrounding area are affected by this type of treatment. When radiation is directed inside the vagina, the ovaries may absorb some radiation also. Radiation directed at the uterus may increase the risk of miscarriage or premature births. If you have had radiation to the pelvic area or to your head, your fertility may be affected. Radiation to the head can damage the pituitary gland, which sends signals to the ovaries to make hormones to trigger ovulation in women.

Cancer surgery and fertility. Surgery is the one common form of cancer treatment as it offers the greatest chance of cure for many types of cancer, especially those that have not spread to other parts of the body. In women, removal of the ovaries, uterus, fallopian tubes, or vagina does affect fertility. For certain women's cancers, a hysterectomy (removal of the uterus) may be part of the treatment. When the ovaries are removed, it is called an *oophorectomy*; one or both ovaries can be removed during the same operation to remove the uterus. Once this surgery is done, a woman cannot carry a child in her uterus. In some selected cases of ovarian cancer or some early cases of cervical cancer, the surgeon will try to do a less aggressive surgical procedure to help preserve a woman's ability to carry a child. Sometimes, the postoperative complications of surgery, like adhesions, can affect fertility. Scarring or fibrosis that blocks the fallopian tubes may affect an embryo or egg from entering into the uterus.

Fertility

Fertility was another big surprise: that chemo-induced menopause could be permanent and I wouldn't be able to have children. Ever. That's a tough one and it is still sinking in. I never in a hundred-thousand years thought I would not be able to have children. If this is an issue for you, be sure to clarify your options before beginning treatment, and get more than one opinion. I didn't do this and I am still angry about it. I should add that I don't think it would have changed the outcome in my case, but I still would like to have been better informed.

Frances S.

82. What are some options to preserve my fertility?

The methods provided in this question describe a few proven options that may help you preserve your fertility. Question 84 is an overview of experimental options. Experimental methods are still under investigation and are being studied in clinical trials and may not be as effective as other options. It is always important to talk with your doctor or healthcare team about which fertility-preserving method is right for you.

Embryo freezing is a proven method for preserving a woman's fertility. Mature eggs are removed from the ovaries, usually in an office-based procedure where eggs are collected using an ultrasound needle that is guided through the upper vagina and uterus, then up into the ovaries. The mature eggs are fertilized with sperm and the resulting embryo is grown and then frozen for future use. Some women may be given hormones to help produce mature eggs and induce **ovulation**. Hormonal stimulation before cancer treatment is

Ovulation

process of egg release from the ovary.

needed to help mature the eggs, so this may not be an option for some women with hormone-sensitive cancers, such as certain breast cancers.

Because embryo freezing requires sperm, many couples who are in stable relationships use this method to store fertilized embryos for future use. Other women may choose an unknown sperm donor or the sperm of a friend to fertilize her eggs. This type of procedure poses concerns for women who do not have a partner. A woman without a partner may have serious doubts about freezing fertilized eggs with sperm from a donor or friend. She may wonder what awaits her in the future. What if she meets someone and marries, but later he has some conflict over what she has done?

Pregnancy rates with thawed embryos range from 10% to 25% per embryo stored. This process can take several weeks and is not be a viable option if you need urgent life-saving cancer treatment.

Fertility-sparing surgical procedures can be used in women who have had ovarian cancer that is classified as borderline, low malignant potential, germ cell tumors, or ovarian sex stroma cell tumors. Sometimes only the one ovary that is affected by the cancer will be removed by the surgeon. This leaves the healthy ovary in place so you are able to ovulate (produce an egg) and possibly become pregnant.

Radical trachelectomy is a new fertility-preserving surgical option for women with early stage cervical cancer. With this method, only the cervix (but not the uterus) is removed for the treatment of early stage cervical cancer. There are several cancer centers in the world that presently offer this procedure. Only a skilled surgeon in the department of gynecology oncology can perform the special surgery. There have been live births reported for women who have undergone this new surgical procedure, but their obstetrical and pre-birth care is often complicated and thus needs to be managed by a high risk perinatology specialist.

Fertility-specific surgeries like the radical trachelectomy are good options only for certain selected patients. These surgeries do not interfere with your cancer treatment. If you are thinking about having a fertility-sparing surgery, talk with a specialized gynecologist oncologist. Discuss the risks, benefits, and likelihood of fertility and pregnancy with the procedure with your gynecological healthcare team.

83. What experimental methods may help preserve fertility?

Egg freezing is an experimental procedure that removes mature eggs from the ovaries and freezes them for future use. At some point in the future, the frozen eggs can be thawed and then fertilized with sperm to produce an embryo. The embryo is then implanted back into a woman's uterus where it will grow and develop. It is unclear how long eggs can be frozen before they are thawed and used. For the best success, more than one egg should be frozen. There are storage fees for frozen eggs, and insurance companies often do not pay for this costly expense. To help the ovaries produce mature eggs, you may be given a hormone called gonadotropin. When the eggs are mature, they are surgically removed from the ovaries. This procedure is done in a doctor's office and can last half an hour. It is typically done with a needle through the pelvis to retrieve the eggs. Egg freezing is a good option if you must start your cancer treatment immediately or for some medical reason you can not or wish not to take hormones that would stimulate the ovaries to produce eggs.

The egg freezing process is experimental and, according to Fertile Hope, pregnancy rates are approximately 3% per egg stored (embryo freezing has pregnancy rates of 10% to 25% per embryo stored). The low success rate with egg freezing, the safety, and efficiency of this method is still not definitively known. About one hundred babies worldwide have been born using this method. There are a few specialized fertility clinics that can do this procedure and some are listed in the Appendix.

Ovarian tissue freezing and transplantation is another medically experimental option for women who wish to attempt to preserve her fertility. With this method, ovarian tissue is surgically removed from the ovaries through small incisions on the abdomen. This procedure uses a very small, video-aided tool called a laparoscope. The ovarian tissue is cut into smaller pieces and then frozen. Usually, after cancer treatment, the tissue can be thawed and transplanted (put back into the woman's body). The ovarian tissue can be placed at many different sites in the woman, including close to the fallopian tubes or in another part of the body like the abdomen or forearm.

Because no fertility drugs are used, ovarian tissue freezing is a good option for women who need to begin immediate cancer treatment. Although this new method is very encouraging for cancer survivors, ovarian tissue freezing and transplantation has recently produced only one live birth.

Ovarian shielding or ovarian transposition is another surgical option for women who will receive radiation therapy to the pelvic area. The ovaries are surgically moved out of the field of the radiation so they do not receive direct radiation. The effectiveness of this method is not known.

GnRH analog treatment is a medication that women can take to temporarily cause menopause (see the introduction to Part 6). These medications can be given in association with chemotherapy. They are frequently used to induce menopause in young women who are undergoing bone marrow transplants due to their underlying cancer. These medications are long-acting injections and can be given on a monthly basis. It is believed that this medication-induced menopause causes the ovaries to be calm (quiescent) and may suffer less damage from cancer treatments. This short-term menopause may reduce damage to immature eggs in the ovaries and lower the risk of infertility. This treatment is experimental, and many scientific studies show no impact of this medication on fertility rates.

84. Are there other options for me to become a parent?

What about natural pregnancy?   It is best to discuss how long you should wait after your cancer therapy before you attempt pregnancy with your medical and surgical oncologists (see Question 81). Every woman's treatment, diagnosis, and prognosis are different. If you do not get pregnant within 12 months of trying to conceive, then you might have a fertility problem. A fertility specialist or reproductive endocrinologist may perform some specialized blood tests to determine whether or not you are fertile. The specialist may do some hormonal evaluations, X-rays, or ultrasound scans of the pelvic area.

According to the American Cancer Society, many patients are advised by their surgical or medical oncologists to wait at least two years before trying to get pregnant. Two years may allow the eggs ample time to recover from the potential damage that might have occurred during treatment. Talk with your doctor about your specific situation.

What about gestational surrogacy? Some women may not be able to become pregnant or carry a pregnancy to term after completing cancer therapy because of severe damage to their pelvic organs. Other women may choose not to become pregnant themselves and opt for surrogacy as a mode to complete their family. Medical concerns, fear of hormonal exposure, or hysterectomy may be other reasons why a woman may choose surrogacy. Although these women may not be able to have a natural pregnancy, they can still have a biological child by using a *gestational surrogate*. Surrogacy involves using another woman's uterus and eggs or just her uterus to carry a child. A gestational surrogate is a healthy female who carries and gives birth to a baby for another person. For example, a fertile surrogate mother may be artificially inseminated with the male partner's sperm. The child will have the genes of the surrogate and the male in this case. In other cases, the egg of the cancer survivor and her partner's sperm are used to create an embryo, which is implanted within the surrogate. In this instance, the embryo that was made using an egg and sperm from the biological parents has no genetic tie or relationship to the host woman. At the completion of the pregnancy (birth), the baby is given to the biological parents. Surrogacy can be a complicated and expensive process. Surrogacy laws vary, so it is important to have a reproductive attorney to help you execute the appropriate legal arrangements with your surrogate.

What about using donor eggs or sperm?   If you do not have healthy eggs or sperm, another option is to use eggs or sperm from a donor. Many agencies specialize in helping you find egg or sperm donors. Egg donors are typically young college-aged women who are extensively screened for medical and psychological traits and usually wish to remain anonymous. You could even ask a close friend or family member who is willing to donate an egg or sperm. If you use an anonymous donor, you may be able to find out many characteristics such as hair and eye color, height, weight, personality, educational history, hobbies, as well as medical, psychiatric, and family histories. Sometimes the agency will even allow you to get the donor's baby picture. Donors of eggs or sperm are screened for sexually transmitted diseases as well as medical and psychological health before being allowed to donate.

If you are thinking about using donor eggs or sperm, discuss your plans with your partner and family. There are many issues to think about, such as whether you will tell your child after he or she grows up. You may even want to talk to a mental health professional who specializes in fertility issues. If you already have a child and need to discuss this issue, children's books are available that can help you with this sensitive topic.

What are donor embryos? Is this experimental option for me?
According to the American Cancer Society's *Fertility and the Cancer Patient* booklet, embryo donation is the newest approach that can allow a couple to experience pregnancy and birth together. Neither parent will have a genetic relationship to the child. Embryo donations usually come from another couple who have used assisted reproductive technology procedures, had children, and have extra embryos that are frozen. When that couple has conceived or for some other reason chooses not to use their extra embryos, they may decide to donate them or allow them to be adopted rather than be destroyed or used for medical stem cell research.

Any woman who has a healthy uterus and can sustain a pregnancy can undergo fertility therapy with donor embryos. Most women who attempt the donor embryo procedure get hormonal treatments to mature the lining of her uterus and ensure the best timing of the embryo transfer. If a woman has ovaries that cannot produce eggs, she will need to receive estrogen and progesterone to prepare her uterus. In this process, the embryos are thawed and transferred to the woman to achieve pregnancy. Following the transfer of the embryos, the woman continues hormone support until blood work shows that the placenta is working on its own, usually around eight to ten weeks. There is no published research on the success rates of embryo donation, so it is important that you research the in vitro fertilization (IVF) success rates in your local reproduction centers. Frozen embryo transfers average around a 19% live birth rate as compared with around 30% live birth rate with fresh embryos.

Can adoption be the answer for me to complete my dream to having a family? For some couples, the only option for children may be adoption. There are many agencies (local, national, and international) that can help you adopt a child. Some agencies specialize in placing children with special needs, older children, or even sibling groups. You should find an agency that is comfortable and has experience working with cancer survivors.

Many adoption agencies require a medical letter from your doctor and many have specific age limits for adoptive parents. The letter from your oncologist usually needs to say that the cancer survivor has a good prognosis. Some may also require that a cancer survivor be cancer-free for at least five years before applying for adoption. Adoption fees vary by the type of adoption you choose. There is a lot of paperwork to complete during the adoption process, and at times it is overwhelming. Many countries allow U.S. citizens to adopt children from their foreign country. Adoption laws vary from country to country, changing often and without notification. Because this is the case, plan to talk to an attorney who specializes in international adoptions. Know the rules and regulations from the country you are adopting from and keep current.

Be sure to choose an adoption agency carefully that can meet your needs and can help you with the application process. Be certain to ask about their policies and procedures as well as their fees before starting the formal application and adoption process. Some couples find it helpful to attend adoption or parenting classes before their adoption. These classes can help you understand the adoption process and allow you to share with other couples in similar situations. The adoption process takes a variable amount of time depending upon the type of adoption you choose. Most adoptions should be accomplished in one to two years. The financial expenditures also vary greatly, ranging from about $3,000 up to as much as $40,000.

85. What are some important questions that I should I ask my doctor about fertility?

The answer to this question is adapted from educational materials from Fertile Hope. If you have any concerns about fertility, discuss them with your doctor and healthcare team. Here are a few questions to help you get started:

- If I choose to have children, will I give the cancer gene to them?
- How will my treatment affect my ability to have children?
- Does my cancer treatment typically cause infertility?
- How will I know if I am infertile after treatment?
- Do I have any options that can help preserve my future fertility?
- What do you think is the best way to preserve my fertility?
- Which option is the safest for me?
- Can my treatment be changed or delayed to preserve my fertility?
- Will any fertility-preserving technique impact my overall survival?

- How long after my cancer treatment should I wait before trying to get pregnant?
- Is pregnancy safe for me after my particular cancer and treatment?
- Where can I find services that offer options to preserve my fertility?

86. What other fertility considerations should I think about after cancer care?

Legal concerns.   With new reproductive techniques, like egg and sperm freezing, donor eggs and sperm, and surrogacy, it is important that you talk to a specialized reproductive attorney. These attorneys can help you understand legal documents as well as your legal and financial rights and obligations. Because you are dealing with complex medical issues, consulting an attorney who is familiar with contracts dealing with reproductive technology is a wise decision. There are also specialized lawyers who work exclusively with adoption services. They can help the birth parents terminate their legal rights and facilitate the adoption process.

Financial concerns.   While many of the tests that diagnose fertility are often covered by insurance, other treatments costs are often not covered. Only a dozen states have laws that require varying amounts of coverage for infertility and in vitro fertilization (IVF) treatments. Many patients are not covered by these laws and others live in states with no or limited insurance coverage. Costs present major barriers for most patients.

According to the American Cancer Society, the first step is to research and decide what treatment might be an option for you, where you can get it, and what the costs are for the best treatment. Some institutions have financial counselors associated with the fertility clinic or medical practice. These experts can guide you through the details about each treatment, its costs, and even specific insurance codes for the services you might need.

At some point, it is wise to sit down and sift through your finances. Consider the money in your bank and retirement accounts, any credit card help, or even financial assistance from family members. Some hospitals and private practices participate in the Fertile Hope financial assistance program, "Sharing Hope," which reduces the costs of fertility preservation for qualifying patients (see the Appendix).

It is hard to think about spending a large amount of money on fertility while you are still dealing with other medical bills related to your cancer illness. Another important barrier is that you may have to act quickly to preserve fertility before your cancer treatment begins. Getting financial help and counseling is a first step and will help you feel less alone as you try to plan for a future beyond cancer.

What about mental health services?   Thinking about your cancer treatment and fertility can make you feel overwhelmed or depressed. These feelings are normal. A mental health professional can help you adjust to your cancer diagnosis and help you deal with your feelings about your fertility. A professional also can help you deal with feelings of guilt, anger, loss, and disability. Your therapist should understand the impact of cancer on fertility and help you think about your parenting options.

The Fertile Help organization and other important resources are listed in the Appendix.

PART 10

Sexual Health

What causes sexual problems in the cancer survivor?

What kinds of treatments exist for my
sexual health management?

Can medication improve my sexual function?

Are sexual devices effective?

Can alternative or complementary medicine
help improve my sex life?

More . . .

Sexual concerns are common for women, and many cancer survivors face the additional issues of a changed self-image, fatigue from their cancer therapies, and mortality. While not life-threatening, not having a healthy and active sex life can affect your entire relationship with your spouse or partner and as well as how you feel about yourself. The ramifications from cancer and its treatment can have a serious affect on your sexual satisfaction and the complaint is extremely prevalent in all women of all ages and for all cancer types. It is important to ask your healthcare professional for help!

Some complain of having a low libido (hypoactive sexual desire disorder), changes in orgasm, or arousal. Sexual pain disorders like **dyspareunia** (pain during intercourse) and vaginismus (reflexive contracture of the pelvic and vaginal muscles) are also prevalent in the female population. Nearly one quarter of those who survived leukemia or Hodgkins disease have distressing sexual dysfunction.

It is important to discuss your sexual concerns with your doctors. An assessment will include a detailed medical and gynecological history, comprehensive general physical and genital examination, and a psychological as well as psychosexual examination. Laboratory tests, such as blood laboratory of various hormones or radiological evaluation, may be appropriate. Sexual status, orientation, and past sexual experience may be important factors to discuss. Patients are encouraged to see a sexual medicine specialist/gynecologist and a sexual psychiatrist or certified sexual **psychologist** for her initial evaluations and follow-up surveillance.

Dyspareunia

pain or discomfort during sexual intercourse.

Psychologist

a degreed, credentialed therapist who councils with patients and their families about emotional and personal matters and can help them make ethical decisions.

Sexual dysfunction is often complex and multidimensional, so an individual's treatment regimen may involve several different approaches. Healthy, satisfying sexual functioning and treatment success are impacted by a variety of factors including medical illnesses, hormonal levels, relationship concerns, partner availability, underlying psychiatric disorders, general medical well being, and cultural and religious behaviors.

87. Am I alone? Do many cancer survivors experience sexual complaints?

According to 2005 statistics from the American Cancer Society, with technological treatments and advancements in diagnostics and therapeutics, an estimated 60% of all cancer survivors will live at least five years after their diagnosis. In 2000, an estimated ten million people were cancer survivors in the United States. Research has shown that sexual complaints that are distressing occur in up to 90% of women who have been diagnosed with cancer. Other studies report the number of women with posttreatment sexual dysfunction ranging from 30% to 100%.

Know that you are not alone if you have some sexual complaints. You may feel embarrassed or ashamed about discussing the issues with your doctors. Once you have discussed your concerns, your physician hopefully should be receptive to helping you with these deeply private issues. But if your doctor is uncomfortable or does not have the technical skills to deal with the sexual side effects of cancer treatment effectively, do not get discouraged. Do not give up! Review the Appendix and find another provider who can help answer all of your concerns, as this ultimately enhances your survivorship quality of life. Sexuality and intimacy are critical for health happiness and feeling connected with both yourself and your partner.

88. What causes sexual problems in the cancer survivor?

A variety of factors can interfere with a woman's sexuality. In addition to her psychological make-up and past experience with intimate relationships (see Questions 73–77) and medications (see Question 81), other cancer treatments may affect how a woman may respond sexually.

Surgery. Operative procedures may change the way your body looks, and some interfere with the nerves in your genital and pelvic area, which are vital to the sexual response cycle. Removal of your reproductive organs may affect your self-esteem and influence how you view yourself as a woman. With extensive surgical resection and radical surgery, women often shift their perceptions of their body and femininity. Large tumor resections that involve extensive physical changes, such as bowel removal, may result in functional changes such as ileostomies, colonostomies, and ileoconduits that may be perceived as embarrassing or ugly (see Question 20).

Prophylactic oophorectomy (risk-reducing bilateral salpingo-oophorectomy, RRBSO)
removal of a woman's eggs and ovaries in an attempt to reduce or eliminate a risk for future cancer.

Women with breast cancer, who have a genetic predisposition for the development of ovarian cancer because of *BRCA* gene mutations, may opt to undergo a **prophylactic oophorectomy** (risk-reducing bilateral salpingo-oophorectomy, RRBSO; see Question 16). Many women who underwent a RRBSO have negative sexual consequences as well as concerns about body image and the development of underlying malignancies. When breast cancer survivors undergo prophylactic mastectomy and/or reconstruction for breast removal, sometimes the breast is not acceptable, which may impact sexual enjoyment and self-image. Surgical scarring after procedures may interfere with extremity mobility, especially with arm movement. Finding a comfortable sexual position may be difficult and challenging.

Radiation therapy. Radiation therapy may cause skin changes like thickening, contractures, or different textures and colors. Other side effects like unexplained fatigue, loss of hair on your head or in the genital area (see Question 63), and gastrointestinal complaints of diarrhea, nausea, and vomiting may all contribute to a lack of interest. Patients and/or their partners may have unfounded fears concerning the myth of being "radioactive." The truth is that you cannot catch radiation nor are you considered radioactive if you have undergone radiation treatment.

Vaginal fibrosis with stiffening and hardening of a shortened vaginal vault can be caused by direct radiation to the vagina. This can seriously impact a woman's capacity for penetrative intercourse and affect her genital pelvic and clitoral sensitivity during sexual activity. Her sexual sensation or orgasms may be less intense than before, so it may take longer to reach the same level of excitement and arousal.

Chemotherapy. Many agents can cause nausea, diarrhea, membrane irritation, and induce premature menopause, which can present as hot flashes and vaginal dryness or atrophy. Loss of hair on the head, eyebrows, eyelashes, and genitals is distressing and affects a female's perception of sexual attractiveness. Chemotherapy-induced early ovarian failure from surgical removal (adjunctive radiation therapy) can cause menopausal symptoms (see Question #48). The symptoms of hot flashes, sleep instability, vaginal dryness, and mood problems also impact desire, sexual interest, and arousal. Vaginal dryness can lead to painful intercourse or penetration.

The use of low-dose serotonin reuptake inhibitors and antihypertensive medications can be used for treatment of distressing hot flashes (see Questions 48, 51–54).

89. How can maintenance hormonal therapies, which keep my cancer under control, impact my sexual function?

Aromatase inhibitors and other medications (like Tamoxifen®, a selective estrogen receptor modulator; SERM) are often used to treat breast cancer and can exacerbate menopausal symptoms. Some research has linked SERMs with vaginal dryness, excessive vaginal discharge, vaginal tenderness, changes in orgasm, and diminished libido. But studies examining the effects of Tamoxifen® on sexual functioning in women are conflicting and inconclusive. The Breast Cancer Prevention Trial states that minor differences in sexual functioning were observed in tamoxifen users versus those not on the medication. In contrast, Mortimer demonstrated no changes in any phase of sexual response cycle for women on tamoxifen.

The aromatase inhibitors (letrozole, anastrozole, and exemestane) block the conversion of testosterone to estrogen and significantly lower the levels of circulating estradiol. While this action is often the objective of breast cancer therapy, it can aggravate menopausal symptoms and cause osteopenia and osteoporosis (see Questions 9 and 10). More scientific trials are needed to specifically address the sexual ramifications of these drugs.

90. What are the psychological changes after cancer that may impact sexual functioning?

Many women report continued feelings of sadness, melancholy, depressive symptoms about their body image, fear of cancer recurrence, and sexuality problems even after becoming cancer-free. Negative sexual experiences that happened in the past (promiscuity, extramarital affairs, and sexually transmitted diseases) may be incorrectly transferred to a patient's genital cancer diagnosis. Underlying psychiatric illnesses and psychopathology combined with depressed moods that can alter self-image all contribute to the development of female sexual dysfunction.

Relationship dynamics change once the woman has a cancer diagnosis. The partner may have their family role reversed. He or she may become the caregiver and/or primary wage earner, which may lead to difficult adjustments to their altered familial roles. Marital and financial tension can be stressful for the couple (see Question 74). Other worries may include the threat of disease recurrence, early death, and bodily disfigurement as well as economic, employment, and insurance concerns.

91. What specific sexual health management therapies can I expect when I seek treatments as a female cancer survivor?

The treatment of female sexual complaints is complex and involves the combined approach of treating the woman's medical issues as well as assessing and treating her sexual psychological issues. Listed here are a variety of therapeutic options that the sexual medicine specialist may perform in order to effectively treat your sexual complaints.

Treatment of systemic illness(es). Cancer survivors often have other underlying medical conditions and illnesses that directly impact on her sexual health and the sexual response cycle. Evaluation and treatment of chronic illnesses, such as uncontrolled hypertension, hypercholesterolemia, and/or an underlying thyroid dysfunction can be simple to identify. Arthritis may impact your mobility and limit finding comfortable sexual positions. Uncontrolled diabetes may influence veins, arteries, and nerves in the genital pelvic region, which may impact blood flow and directly affect excitement (vasocongestion and pelvic engorgement).

Underling genital infections like candida (yeast), bacterial vaginosis, and *Trichomoniais* should be treated. Often, sexual specialists include screening, such as a complete blood profile to rule out underlying anemia, complete lipid profiles, glucose screening, and prolactin levels. Estrogen and progesterone as well as other hormonal profiles are typically measured, too.

In the acute crisis of cancer care, sometimes pre-existing medical illnesses can be neglected. So, treating any underlying chronic medical illnesses not only improves your general physical and mental well being but may improve your sexuality as well.

Medications.   Most classes of drugs can affect the female sexual response cycle and cause sexual problems. Many antidepressants and antihypertensive medications can change sexual desire, arousal, and orgasm. Ask your physicians to check pharmacologic guides to identify potential offending agents and consider substituting another drug. Sexual pharmacology textbooks are available for quick and easy reference and you can check the Internet as well (be sure to review the National Institutes of Health and respected medical school Web sites; see the Appendix).

Some young women on birth control pills complain of sexual issues. The biochemistry in these tablets may decrease free bioavailable testosterone, which has been linked to sexual desire and interest. Simply switching these women to an alternative form of contraception may improve sexual functioning.

The medical treatment of sexual dysfunction often includes changing medication regimens, altering dosing and/or time intervals, or switching to a new drug. Never abruptly stop any prescribed medication without first consulting with your prescribing physician. There may be a good alterative or one that causes fewer or less intense side effects. Some studies show that women who suffer from sexual dysfunction as a result of their antidepressant medications (like serotonin reuptake inhibitors) may benefit from a trial of Phosphodiesterase inhibitors such as Viagra®, Cialis®, or Levitra®.

Structured sexual exercises and behavioral modification. Patients with sexual complaints are always encouraged to make lifestyle modifications that will enhance and improve quality of life. A well-balanced nutritious diet combined with an active aerobic exercise plan is vital. Stopping the use of tobacco and illicit drugs combined with minimizing alcohol consumption is also encouraged. If fatigue is a problem, take frequent naps and plan sexual intimacy when you are well rested. Very often, incorporating time and stress management skills into scheduling time for sex and intimacy is helpful. Sexual intimacy needs to become a priority for you and your partner. Set limits with other commitments such as employment, social responsibilities, and family obligations. Technological machinery like cellular telephones, Blackberries, pagers, and computer laptops, although helpful in the workplace, often interfere with private time. If you are preoccupied with these devices, you maybe suffering from a "soft addiction." Soft addictions can limit intimacy and take away from time spent together as a couple. Limit use of these devices to a specific time frame and monitor your time spent on them so that it does not hinder sexual intimacy and interpersonal communication.

Similarly, patients can be given specific sexually structured tasks to identify and help with specific sexual complaints. Some examples of behavior modification sexual techniques include:

- Erotic reading (Try reading an erotic novel in a quiet, relaxed place!)
- Sensate focusing (concentrate on your physical sensations)

- Squeeze–stop technique (alternately tightening your pelvic muscles and relaxing)
- Guided imagery (imagining a particular scenario)
- Relaxation techniques (breathing exercises)
- Exploration of sexual fantasies (using props or mental imagery)
- Self stimulation (masturbation) exercises

Many patients are assigned homework in the form of sexual exploration. These may include non-genital touching, self stimulation exercise, and other sexual exercises to improve and enhance your sexual self-esteem. Patients and their partners are educated through the use of open discussions concerning alternate forms of sexual expression like mutual massage, intimate fondling and caressing, or manual, digital, or oral and anal stimulation. Let your imagination be your guide.

Patients and their partners may be encouraged to engage in alternative sexual positions. Most couples engage in intercourse in the missionary position which may facilitate deep penetration. But this position can be very painful for the woman who has a shortened vagina in association with vaginal and vulvar atrophy. Sexual intercourse in alternative positions may include side-to-side (spooning) or female superior positions, which may help limit deep pelvic thrusting and minimize vaginal discomfort during penetration. Other sexual positions encourage direct clitoral stimulation, which greatly facilitates arousal in many women. If movement and mobility are issues (e.g., chronic arthritis, bone and/or joint illness), pillows or down comforters can be used to help create a comfortable sexual situation.

Tantra

ancient Indian spiritual tradition and belief system with the premise that sexuality is tied into personal energy and is capable of changing us if we submit to our primal sexual desires while maintaining control and heightening spiritual awareness. When incorporated into lovemaking, tantra ultimately intensifies the sexual dynamic or consciousness between couples.

Tantra is the ancient Indian spiritual tradition and belief system that sexuality is tied into personal energy. Practicing Tantra, according to Tantric experts, is capable of changing us if we submit to our primal sexual desires while maintaining control and heightening spiritual awareness. When incorporated into lovemaking, the techniques ultimately intensify the sexual dynamic or consciousness between couples as they fully experience their sensual and sexual energy together. Sexual enhancement, pleasuring, living consciously, and the various postures of lovemaking are important tenets of Tantra. The union of the *yin and yang* (the male and female) expands the dimensions of sexuality, and through the control of orgasms, feelings of intimacy and connectedness with your partner are ultimately enhanced.

Sex therapy specialists are located in most areas of the United States. Drs. Lana Holstein and David Taylor offer an excellent sexual intimacy workshop located at the Life Balance Spa Miraval in Arizona. Through lectures and workshops, their program teaches couples to reconnect sexually, thus reclaiming sexual enrichments and satisfaction by exploring sexual pleasure and passion. Further information about their programs is on the Internet (http://www.miravalresort.com).

Pain. Complaints of chronic discomfort or pain can influence a woman's sexual response and limit her interest and enjoyment of sexual activity. When pain is at low level and fatigue minimum, sexual expression should be encouraged. Techniques such as warm soaks and physical therapy help loosen tense muscles. Guided imagery, meditation, deep-muscle relaxation, and avoidance of exhaustion are options that should be explored. Specifically trained pain management specialists can be consulted to adjust or reduce opioid regimens, add adjunctive or alternative **analgesics**, and modify existing dosing schedules, which may lessen fatigue while maintaining sufficient pain relief.

Sexual education.   Women often are not educated about sexual responsiveness and genital anatomy. Understanding your genital anatomy will help you know your normal physiological response and how arousal occurs. Examine you genitals with the aid of a hand held mirror and with the assistance of a healthcare professional. Do you know where the clitoral tissue is located?

Bibliotherapy consists of many take-home items, such as pamphlets, books, videos, and other visual aids, which provide educational reinforcement and serve as a future reference. There are many widely published resources available. Many women may opt to search the Internet when seeking information concerning the treatment of her sexual problems. The Women's Sexual Health Foundation, The International Society for the Study of Women's Sexual Health (ISSWSH), North American Menopause Society (NAMS), and the American College of Obstetricians and Gynecologists (ACOG) are all organizations that maintain wonderful information on their Web sites concerning sexual health and sexual education. They also provide medical information about the latest updates on female sexual therapeutics. For the female cancer survivor, the American Cancer Society's booklet, *Cancer and Sexuality* is an excellent patient reference guide. It provides factual information and helpful suggestions to maintain and improve your sexual functioning (contact your oncologist or see the Appendix).

Analgesics
type of medication used to treat pain.

Sexual Health

Psychosexual therapy and counseling. Because women's sexual complaints are a complex phenomenon and situational issues are a fundamental part of the diagnosis, a comprehensive treatment regime would not be complete without appropriate sexual counseling and therapy. Sexual complaints are best treated by a certified sexual therapist who is educated and trained to deal with patients with sexual complaints. These specialists are qualified to deal with psychosexual issues that include body image, changes in intimacy, sexuality, self-esteem, and mood. Issues about the ramifications of cancer and its therapy are covered, too. You may also need marital, individual, couples, and/or group therapy, depending on the need and specific complaint. In general, most patients can benefit from brief psychosexual interventions that include education, counseling/support, and symptom management. Psychotherapist and psychologists can be extremely effective when vaginal dilators are prescribed for the treatment of vaginismus, where a woman's muscles in her vagina close tightly almost involuntarily. Close contact with the medical clinician and psychosexual therapist can help alleviate your sexual symptoms. Frequent visits to your healthcare professional are often needed to help with vaginismus.

Local and national support organizations like the American Association for Sex Education, Counseling and Treatment (AASECT; http://www.aasect.org) and Association of Reproductive Health Professionals (ARHP) can provide further information and support to help patients achieve greater comfort with these issues, both within their relationships and families and within themselves.

92. What pharmacologic interventions can improve my sexual function?

Systemic and local estrogen replacement remains key in the management of female sexual dysfunction. Estrogen is one of many important hormones that are necessary for sexual function in women. Central arousal and peripheral and pelvic sexual response are dependant on estrogen levels and in some instances testosterone levels as well. Systemic hormonal replacement can be achieved with a variety of products either taken orally or transdermally (through a skin patch).

For women who have an intact uterus, the standard of care is to add a progestin agent to the regime; this prevents endometrial hyperplasia and endometrial cancer. With the emerging data from the Woman's Health Initiative study, there are growing concerns about hormones and potential associated risks of cardiovascular events or breast cancer (see Question 49). Risks and benefit profiles should be discussed with your healthcare and sexual medicine specialist.

Estrogen has many effects on the urogenital system. It not only promotes epithelial cell maturation and proliferation, increases vascularity and blood flow, but also stimulates glandular secretions. A decrease of estrogen causes decreased vasocongestion (increased blood supply to the genitals), increased atrophic vaginitis, and can lead to dyspareunia (painful intercourse) and possibly a reactive lowered desire. The use of local vaginal estrogen (creams, rings, and tablets) for the treatment of vaginal atrophy is widely accepted. Many products are minimally absorbed (Estring® and Vagifem® vaginal tablets). Premarin® and Estrace® cream are other hormonal products which maybe used for the vagina and the vulvar tissues. Many women find these products especially soothing to the irritated pelvic area. Some sexual health providers prefer to prescribe local 17â-estradiol tablet, (Vagifem®), which is minimally absorbed into the systemic circulation. Vaginally administered estrogens in small topically-applied doses can be well absorbed. Patients say that the tablets are also easy to use, less messy than cream preparations, and technically easier to insert than estrogen rings. It is important to recognize that estrogen use is not without risks or complications. Some of the side effects include possible blood clots (thromboembolic events), increased heart problems (cardiovascular events), an increase in breast cancer, and increased endometrial cancer if unopposed with a progestin. The long term safety data on minimally absorbed local vaginal estrogen products used in cancer patients remains to be further studied. Talk with your clinician to analyze which one may be the right solution for you and your partner.

93. What is testosterone replacement and how is it linked with women's sexuality?

Replacement of testosterone in females remains controversial and many researchers are still unconvinced about any direct linkage between testosterone and female sexual health. The data are confusing and conflicting. **Female androgen insufficiency** syndrome is a medical condition characterized by blunted or decreased motivation, persistent fatigue, and a decreased sense of personal well being that is identified by insufficient plasma estrogen, low circulating

Female androgen insufficiency

a syndrome characterized by blunted or diminished motivation, persistent fatigue, and a decreased sense of personal well being that may be characterized by insufficient plasma estrogen, low circulating bioavailability testosterone, and low sexual desire (libido).

bioavailability of testosterone, and low sexual desire (libido). Other potential symptoms include bone loss, decreased muscle strength, and changes in cognition or memory. Bone density may also be affected.

The North American Menopause Society published a comprehensive position statement in September 2005 in its inclusive review of testosterone use, which included monitoring, safety, and replacement guidelines and dosages for postmenopausal women. At the time of this book's publication, there is no U.S. FDA-approved androgen product available for women. The use of male products or bioidentical products should be used with caution and more long-term safety data is warranted. It is interesting to note that in Europe the testosterone patch Intrinsa® has been recently approved and will be released shortly.

Very high levels of testosterone may have several potential serious side effects including, but not limited to, increased facial and body hair growth (hirsuitism), weight gain, abnormal enlargement of the clitoris (clitoromegaly), hair loss (alopecia), changes in lipid profiles, and liver or hematological changes. Women who have taken testosterone supplements also have reported emotional changes. The safety of androgen in the cancer population has not been adequately studied. There is a concern that the testosterone can be converted or aromatized to estrogen, which may reactivate, promote, or stimulate tumor growth. The new testosterone transdermal matrix patch (Intrinsa®) may prove to be promising for libido issues; however, further randomized controlled trials that examine long-term safety data are warranted.

Some of the testosterones successfully used in women include oral methyltestosteone, transdermal testosterone, topical testosterone prioprionate cream 2%, testosterone gel, and oral dehydroepiandrosterone (DHEA). There are also medications that combine estrogen and an androgen component (Estratest® and Estratest HS®–half strength). A woman who is taking testosterone off label in an effort to have increased desire or for libido issues should be under the care of a sexual medicine specialist and should have her blood laboratory values monitored closely. The blood, lipid, and liver should be monitored and any side effects reported immediately to her clinician.

94. Are there other medications that have been used in women for the treatment of sexual complaints?

The following list includes many, but not all, of the latest medications.

Phosphodiesterase inhibitors (Viagra®, Levitra®, Cialis®, and Tadalafil®) are medications that have been approved for the treatment of erectile dysfunction in men. Numerous attempts have been made to show an efficacy in women, but most fail to show any significant benefit in randomized clinical trials. The proposed mechanism of action is that the medication relaxes the clitoral and vaginal smooth muscle. Some potential side effects include headache, uterine contractions, dizziness, hypotension, myocardial infarction (heart attack), stroke, and sudden death. Exciting emerging data may support their use in women who suffer from sexual complaints as a result of hypertension, diabetes, neural and vascular disease, or selective serotonin reuptake inhibitor (SSRI) use.

Alprostadil (Alista®) is a prostaglandin E_1 component that is not FDA approved for the treatment of female sexual dysfunction. However, this topical medication can be applied to the pelvic genital area twice a day assumedly to relax arterial smooth blood vessels, causing vasodilatation and increased sensitivity and sexual arousal. Possible side effects include pain to the genitals, lowered blood pressure, and possible temporary fainting (syncope).

Bupropion (Wellbutrin®) is a non-SSRI antidepressant, dopamine agonist, which has recently been touted as the antidepressant medication with the least sexual side effects. This medication is a weak blocker of the brain chemicals serotonin and norepineherine uptake and is commonly used in smoking cessation programs. A typical trial of this medication includes a starting dose of 75 mg that can be increased gradually. Precautions include insomnia, nervousness, and mild-to-moderate increases in blood pressure as well as a risk of lowering seizure threshold.

Three other medications that are still under investigation include:

- *Flibanserin*, a 5-HT1A agonist/5-HT2 antagonist (Boehrringer Ingelheim). Some of the mild side effects include nausea, dizziness, fatigue, sleeplessness, and possibly increased bleeding if on an NSAIDs or ASA. It is very promising for the treatment of female sexual desire disorder.

- *Tibolone* (Organon) is not available in the United States. It has been shown to reduce hot flashes, increase bone mineral density, and women report that it decreases vaginal dryness. The drug does improve desire, not sexual function. There are some medical concerns regarding the lipid metabolism, hemostasis, and long-term cardiovascular and cancer risks.
- *Bremelanotide* (PT 141; Palatin Technologies) is a melanocortin receptor agonist for the treatment of female sexual complaints. A Phase 2A pilot clinical study looked at this medication in premenopausal women diagnosed with female sexual dysfunction (FSD) and it has shown encouraging results.

Before taking any of these medications, it is crucial to discuss their potential benefits and risks with your oncologist or clinician.

95. What non-hormonal and non-medication regimes can I use to help with my sexual function?

Because hormones do pose serious risks and other medications have some side effects, women may opt to use other types of treatment to help their sexual function. Some helpful sexual products include vaginal moisturizers and lubricants.

What are vaginal moisturizers? The liberal use of local non-medicated, non-hormonal vaginal moisturizers (Replens® or vitamin E suppositories) can provide relief for the symptoms of vaginal atrophy. These agents are recommended for use two or three times weekly. Women should wear a light pad when using vitamin E suppositories because it may stain undergarments. Feminease® is another type of moisturizer and it claims to be all-natural. Another option is Moist Again®.

What are vaginal lubricants? The use of water-based vaginal lubricants with intercourse is also encouraged when vaginal dryness and atrophy are diagnosed. However, vaginal lubricants that contain microbicides, perfumes, coloration, and flavors may irritate the sensitive atrophic vaginal mucosa. Lubricate all surfaces as part of foreplay and be sure to keep lubricant handy in case more is needed. Lubricants may be water- or silicone-based. Be certain to use a lot of lubricant when attempting intercourse if you are in the middle of treatment for vaginal atrophy or dryness.

Some brands of water-based lubricants include Astroglide®, Liquid Silk®, GV Slip Inside®, Hydrasmooth®, Sensua Organic®, Probe®, and KY Jelly®. Silicone-based lubricants are Wet Platinum® and Eros Women®.

96. What are some common sexual devices?

There are many sexual accessories that a woman can purchase to help stimulate the genitals. Some enhance pleasure while others are part of a complicated sexual medicine treatment plan. Let your imagination be your guide and explore your sexual fantasies with your mate.

What is a vaginal dilator? For women who have undergone pelvic surgery, suffer from vaginal shortening or vaginal narrowing, or have scar tissue that interferes or prevents penetration and causes vaginal pain, her pelvic discomfort often makes her avoid sexual behavior.

Vaginal dilators may be prescribed as part of their sexual rehabilitation regime. These dilators are graded-size vaginal inserts usually made of plastic or silicone. Dilators are often used to facilitate lengthening and widening of the vagina. They may also be used to help stretch the vaginal scar tissue that may have contributed to pain and discomfort during vaginal intercourse. Dilators can be used on a regular basis and with water- or hormone-based lubricants. Suggested schedules range from once daily for 10 to 15 minutes or at least three times weekly. Several studies report that ongoing supportive behavioral therapy is instrumental for continued compliance.

How do you use a vaginal dilator? Using the vaginal dilator can help expand the vagina and help stretch radiation changes of tissue fibrosis (such as hardening of the vaginal wall tissue) that may have been caused from cancer therapy. Prepare yourself and your environment for dilator therapy. Make certain you will have privacy by either locking your door or working with your dilator when you will not be interrupted. Many clinicians advise women to use their dilators in the morning hours just before starting the day for several reasons. At the end of a long busy day with work, family, and social obligations, many women believe that it is too time-consuming to do the dilator therapy. Too often fatigue and rest supersede sexual rehabilitation. Another reason to do dilator therapy in the morning is that after completion, you can jump in the shower and clean off if the lubricant was messy and/or has resulted in any vaginal leakage. The dilator should be inserted into the vagina with a generous amount of water-based lubricant (see Question 95). You should lie on your back, bend your knees, and spread your knees apart. With gentle pressure, the vaginal dilator should be inserted into the vagina as deeply as possible while still maintaining some comfort. You should leave the dilator in place for ten to fifteen minutes while remaining on your back. It is often helpful to be distracted by other activities while the dilator is in place, like reading a book or watching television. After removing the dilator, it is important to wash it with soap and warm water, dry it with a clean towel, and store it in a safe secure place (adapted from MSKCC patient education materials).

What is the Eros Clitoral Stimulator®? This is a sexual device (Urometrics) that may be prescribed for patients who have had cervical cancer and other pelvic cancers, such as rectal and vaginal cancers. It is battery operated and has a vacuum suction that attaches to the clitoral area. It is presumed to help facilitate vasocongestion in the clitoral tissue. Preliminary data showed promising results that this device may be helpful in combating arousal difficulties after cervical cancer therapy. It is costly and is available by prescription. Insurance plans vary as to whether they will cover the expense.

What about commercially available vibrators or self-stimulators? Vibrators come in a variety of shapes, sizes, and colors. These sexual devices can be helpful for women who may need extra vibratory stimulation in both the sensitive erotic areas of the vagina and clitoris. Vibrators have proven useful during self-stimulatory behavior and can also be used during sexual foreplay. They are available at local pharmacies, the Internet, and at local sexual paraphernalia shops. Self-stimulators can be used with water-based lubricants. It is important to keep them clean; wash them with soap and warm water using a sponge or cloth and rinse well. Store in a clean place.

Vibrators can be used alone as part of self-erotic exploration and sexual play or as part of your sexual repertoire with your partner or lover. Generally, sexual massagers can be used both internally and externally to enhance stimulation, arousal, and pleasure. You can stimulate the labia, vaginal tissue, and clitoral tissue, and even enhance testicular or penile stimulation for your partner. If you share your sexual toys then it is important to cleanse them in between person use.

One Web site (http://drugstore.com) offers home delivery of sexual accessories in a discrete manner and you will not receive any unwanted emails or mailings. One new self-stimulator, the Adonis®, created by the sexual expert Dr. Laura Berman, has gained popularity because it actively stimulates both the clitoral region and the vaginal G spot. The electronic stimulation device called Slight touch® is a battery operated, over-the-counter device that applies electrodes to the top of the foot above the ankles and above the buttocks to stimulate nerve pathways to the genital areas. The Vivelle® device is a battery-operated external clitoral stimulation device that is worn on the fingers and may help orgasm. It is used with a special lubricant and is available over-the-counter. Some other very popular female sexual devices include The Rabbit®, and The Pocket Rocket®. Both are extremely popular among women and have been reported to enhance sexual stimulation and orgasmic intensity.

97. Can alternative and complementary medicine improve my sex life?

Women have tried many nonconventional sexual enhancers and therapeutics in order to facilitate treatment for sexual function complaints and arousal disorders. Many products claim to improve sexual function and some alternative therapies may contain dangerous ingredients. They are also known to have serious and detrimental side effects. There are limited scientifically-proven databases containing results of randomized control trial studies that demonstrate beneficial use of these substances for alleviating sexual dysfunction. In fact, many have some concerning side effects and can interact with prescription medications. It is best to consult with your physician as to whether or not a particular product is right for you. This list highlights a few of the more frequently used products.

DHEA. Some studies show that a low level (50 mg/day) of dehydroepiandroster (DHEA) can improve the frequency of sexual thoughts, sexual interest, and sexual satisfaction over a placebo. It can be prescribed at a starting dosage of 50 mg/day and has shown to increase libido in some women. Caution should be used with this because it can increase androgens, decrease high density lipoprotein (HDL), decrease sex-hormone binding globulin (SHBG), and high levels of DHEA are correlated with increased risk of cardiovascular disease. Caution should be used as these products are not monitored by the FDA and label claims may not accurately reflect the actual DHEA content in the product.

Avlimil is an herbal 756-milligram per day supplemental tablet consisting of sage leaf, red raspberry leaf, capsicum pepper, licorice root, bayberry fruit, damiana leaf, valeriana root, ginger root, black cohosh root, isoflavones, kudzu root extract, and red clover extract (see http://www.avlimil.com for the comprehensive details). Sage, kudzu, red clover licorice, and black cohosh are known to have estrogenic effects and were used in the past for the treatment of menopausal hot flashes and other symptoms. Damiana leaf has been said to act as an aphrodisiac, but no scientific data support this claim. The product package insert states that it is a nonsynthetic, nonhormonal supplement that does not contain estrogen, progesterone, testosterone, or steroid hormones. However the fine print of the labeling states: "If estrogen levels are low, isoflavones are reported to act as 'weak estrogens.'" Avlimil is presumed to increase sexual satisfaction by increasing genital pelvic blood flow and promoting relaxation. A small, unpublished trial of less than fifty women claims a positive effect on female sexual response. Side effects can include minor irritation to stomach upset.

Xzite is a daily dietary supplement that claims to stimulate the brain centrally at the level of the medulla oblongata, which will facilitate mood and increase blood flow to the female genital pelvis. Its ingredients include ligusticum, acathopanax, and chrysanthemum. One unpublished study showed improvement in vaginal lubrication, clitoral sensation, orgasmic satisfaction, and sexual desire.

Arginmax (www.arginimax.com) is a daily supplement that claims to enhance a woman's sexual response by promoting genital pelvic blood flow and promoting relaxation. It is a blend of L-arginine, Korean ginseng, ginkgo biloba, damiana, calcium, iron, and 14 vitamins (for more information, see http://www.arginimax.com). The product claims to increase smooth muscular relaxation, promote vascular dilatation, and enhance clitoral engorgement and vaginal lubrication. One very small published study showed an improvement in sexual desire, clitoral sensation, and frequency of orgasms; satisfaction; and increased frequency of sexual intercourse. Larger ongoing clinical trials are presently being conducted.

Libidol is another daily supplement that consists of sage leaf, red raspberry leaf, kudzu root extract, red clover extract, capsicum pepper, licorice root, bayberry fruit, damiana leaf, valerian root, ginger root, black cohosh root, L-arginine, horny goat weed, and wild oats. Its claims of improving female sexual dysfunction have not been scientifically proven.

Other nutriceuticals and **botanicals** include avena sativa, catuaba, St Johns wart, red sage, angus castus, bethroot, calendula, black cohash, burdock, dong quai, deer antler, eurycoma longifolic, chasie berry, comfrey, fenugreek, evening primrose oil, fennel, licorice root, red clover, raspberry leaf, ginger, horny goat weed, rhino horn, royal jelly, saw palmetto, wild yam zinc, koala nut, maca, and ginseng.

What about diet or nutrition to improve sexual function? Although patients try many different foods, such as chocolate, ginseng, oysters, and popular sexual-enhancing diets, to facilitate improved sexual function, none have been shown in randomized clinical trials to be beneficial for correcting female sexual complaints. Some of the more popular diets include:

- *The Orgasmic Diet:* This includes avoidance of anti-depressants, coffee, tea, caffeine, soft drinks, cigarettes, herbal stimulants, ginkgo, ginseng, and adds high dose vitamins: a multivitamin with vitamin E (400mg), vitamin C, 6-g fish oil [omega-3], calcium

Botanicals
plants or plant parts valued for their medicinal properties; includes herbal products that are commonly prepared as a tea, an extract, or a tincture.

(100 mg), magnesium (400 mg), zinc (15 mg), and slow release iron. Women are encouraged to maintain a low carbohydrate diet, perform Kegel pelvic exercises (see Question 59), and consume one ounce of dark chocolate daily.

- *The Testosterone Diet* consists of nuts, olive oil, canola oil, peanut butter, turnips, broccoli, cabbage, mustard greens, Brussels sprouts, radishes, collard greens, watercress, and bok choy. Avoid all alcohol and maintain good sleep patterns and regular aerobic exercise.

- *The Gladiator Diet* includes weight lifting exercise and a diet void of alcohol, any sweets, and processed foods while ingesting a balanced diet consisting of 33% each of calories from carbohydrates, fats, and proteins.

What are aphrodisiacs?   Aphrodisiacs have been heralded since ancient times as a way to enhance sexual performance and improve desire. However, scientific and medical data are lacking to advocate their use. Some of the more commonly accepted food aphrodisiacs include oysters, lobster, mussels, horseradish, lettuce, carrots, celery, caffeine, mustard seeds, radishes, wine, champagne, truffles, and spices (nutmeg, cayenne pepper, cinnamon, coriander, basil, clover, cardamom, and honey).

Chocolate is often associated with romance, apology, and seductive gifts. It does contain biogenic amines, tyramine, phenylethamine (PEA; the so-called "love drug"), methylxanthines, and cannabinoid-like fatty acids. It is also thought to enhance or promote sensuality and improve sexual function or virility. Unfortunately, a recent study published in the *Journal of Sexual*

Medicine failed to find an association between the consumption of chocolate with sexual function.

98. What are topical formulations that can enhance sexual arousal or function?

There are many lotions that can be massaged into the skin and purport to be sexually enhancing. Check with your oncologist as to the brands that may be right for you.

Zestra® is an herbal topical feminine arousal liquid marketed as a sexual enhancer (for more information: http://www.zestraforwomen.com). It is a blend of borage seed oil, evening primrose oil, angelica root extract, coleus forskohlii extract, ascorbyl palmitate, dl-alpha tocopherol, and natural fragrances. One very small study showed a decrease in sexual complaints. Zestra can increase vaginal and clitoral warmth for up to 30 to 45 minutes after a single application, facilitating sexual arousal and ultimately leading to increased pleasure. Mild genital burning has been reported after application in this study. Borage and evening primrose oils can be metabolized in the skin to increase blood flow and nerve conduction.

Viacreme® is a topical, water-based lotion with menthol and L-arginine (for more information: http://www.viacreme-viacream-viagra.com) that is advertised as a product to enhance sexual responsiveness in the genital area. It is also thought to increase genital warming and clitoral sensitivity. To date, no human studies have been conducted to prove the efficacy of this product and many patients complain of severe genital burning and irritation after application.

Other agents: Less popular agents with various components include: Passion Drops, Lioness, Vaso rect Ultra, Emerita, Natural Curves, and OMY. Dream Cream is another nonprescription vaginal cream that is marketed as a sexual enhancer. It is odorless, colorless, and combines with your own lubrication to help stimulate female genital arousal and blood flow. Its primary ingredient is L-arginine. It should be rubbed into the clitoral region to enhance orgasm approximately 10 minutes before sexual intimacy. It does not contain any hormones nor does it contain menthol, which can be irritating to some women. The cream is not FDA-approved nor have there been any rigorous scientific studies to prove its efficacy.

99. When do I need outside consultation for the treatment of my sexual complaints?

Referral for an evaluation by a subspecialist may be appropriate for certain clinical conditions. Consultants may include: oncologists, social services providers, nutritionists, exercise therapists, and psychiatrists. A list of clinicians and ancillary staff who are sensitive to sexual issues should be readily available for patients who take part in sexual rehabilitation programs. Providers need to reassure patients and their partners that even at the end of life when intercourse may not be feasible, intimacy and emotional closeness should be encouraged. The giving and receiving of sexual pleasure can be accomplished with sensual massage; oral and digital non-coital stimulation with gentle caressing can be very pleasurable.

Sexual complaints are often complex and often require the joint treatment effort from a medical professional and a psychotherapist who are trained in the field of sexual medicine (see Questions 90 and 91). Quality of life, intimacy, and improved sexual function are vital aspects of a woman's life. Sexual concerns are at the forefront of importance for both clinicians and patients. Sexual concerns and dysfunctions during many aspects of the lifecycle or following cancer therapy are often overlooked. The goal of a comprehensive sexual health evaluation and the resulting therapy is to promote sexual health by fostering open communication, provide anticipatory guidance, and validate normalcy with respect to sexual thoughts and feelings. Individual treatment plans are created and implemented by the sexual healthcare professional team to educate patients so they can enjoy fulfilling intimacy and sexual intercourse.

100. Where can I go to learn more about the issues discussed in this book?

The resources listed in the Appendix are what I recommend to my oncology patients during the course of their oncology treatment. Accessing them can provide you with a foundation of organizations, information, and sources that I hope will help you in your survivorship journey.

Appendix

Organizations

American Cancer Society
http://www.cancer.org
(800) ACS-2345

Association of Cancer Online Resources
http://www.acor.org

Cancer Information Network
http://www.thecancer.info

CancerSource
http://www.cancersource.com

Cancer Care, Inc.
http://www.cancercare.org
(800) 813-4673

Centers for Disease Control and Prevention
http://www.cdc.gov/cancer
(888) 842-6355

National Breast Cancer Coalition
http://www.natlbcc.org
(800) 622-2838

National Cancer Information Center
(800) ACS-2345

National Cancer Institute (NCI) Cancer Information Service
http://cancer.gov
(800) 4-CANCER

Survivorship Resources

Cancer Survivorship Network
http://www.acscsn.org

Livestrong®, Lance Armstrong Foundation
http://www.livestrong.org
(512) 236-8820

National Coalition for Cancer Survivorship (NCCS)
http://www.canceradvocacy.org/
(877) 622-7937

National Comprehensive Cancer Network
Has guidelines for management of various cancer-related
    symptoms including fatigue.
http://www.nccn.org
(888) 909-NCCN

People Living with Cancer
Sponsored by the American Society of Clinical Oncologists
    (ASCO)
http://www.peoplelivingwithcancer.org
(703) 797-1914

Specific Groups

Breast Cancer
http://www.breastcancer.org

Colon Cancer
http://www.preventcancer.org/colorectal
http://www.cancer.org
(877) 35-COLON

Gynecologic Cancer Foundation
http://www.wcn.org/gcf
(312) 644-6610

National Council on Aging
http://www.ncoa.org

National Institute of Health
http://www.nih.gov

The Mautner Project for Lesbians with Cancer
http://www.mautnerproject.org
(202) 332-5536

The Susan G. Komen Breast Cancer Foundation
http://www.komen.org
(800) IM-AWARE (800-462-9273)

The Wellness Community
http://help@wellness-community.org
http://www.wellness-community.org
(888) 793-WELL

The Women's Cancer Network
http://www.wcn.org

Nutrition

Limited reliable information concerning nutrients, vitamins, and herbs is available for the cancer survivor. Information found on the Internet often is confusing and contradictory. It is therefore important that you educate yourself before taking any type of product. Some of the best sources for state-of-the-art accepted medical information include:

Memorial Sloan Cancer Center: http://www.mskcc.org/
M. D. Anderson Cancer Center:
    http://www.mdanderson.org/topics/complementary
National Center for Complementary and Alternative Medicine,
    National Institutes of Health: http://www.nccam.nih.gov

Appendix

Pap Smear Information

American Social Health Association: http://www.ashastd.org

American Cancer Society: http://www.cancer.org

American College of Obstetricians and Gynecologists:
    http://www.acog.org

Centers for Disease Control and Prevention: http://www.cdc.gov

Women's Cancer Network: http://www.wcn.org

Vitamins, Dietary Supplements, Minerals, and Botanical Information

American Botanical Council

http://www.herbalgram.org

(512) 926-4900

American Institute for Cancer Research

This organization supports research on diet and nutrition, and
    how it can prevent and treat cancer.

http://www.aicr.org

(800) 843-8114

**Center for Food Safety and Applied Nutrition of the U.S. Food
and Drug Administration**

http://www.cfsan.fda.gov

(888)-SAFEFOOD

Memorial Sloan Kettering Cancer Center

About herbs, botanicals, and other products.

http://www.mskcc.org

National Center for Complementary and Alternative Medicine

http://www.nccam.nih.gov

(888) 644-6226

**Office of Dietary Supplements of the National Institute of
Health**

http://www.dietary-supplements.info.nih.gov

Smoking Cessation

American Cancer Society
Quit Smoking Program
(800) 227-2345

American Lung Association
http://www.lungusa.org

Center for Disease Control and Prevention
http://www.cdc.gov/tobacco/how2quit.htm

Mayo Clinic
Nicotine Dependence Center
http://www.mayoclinic.org/stop-smoking/

Fatigue and Pain Management

Cancer Fatigue
http://www.cancerfatigue.org

The National Pain Foundation
http://www.painconnection.org

Menopause

North American Menopause Association
http://www.menopause.org

American College of Obstetricians and Gynecologists
http://www.acog.org

Other Helpful Resources

Hair

Raquel Welch Sheer Indulgence authorized Starpro™ retailer
http://www.rwstarpro.com
(800) 663-3758

Garments

Ladies First

Wholesale manufacturer offers post-mastectomy products including bras, camisoles, and active wear.
http://www.info@ladiesfirst.com
(800) 663-3758

Lucy's Breast Forms

This store offers many different products for the breast cancer
survivor including bras, enhancers, and attachable nipples.
http://www.lucys.net
(866) 264-9500

A Fitting Experience

A post-mastectomy boutique that sells bras, camisoles, swimsuits,
and wigs. They also have an array of turbans, nightgowns, and
camisoles for the breast cancer survivor.
http://www.mastectomyshop.com
(888) 966-7068

The New You Mastectomy Boutique, LLC

A wide selection of mastectomy products is available by brand.
http://www.newyouboutique.com
(888) 737-2511

Nicola Jane

This Europe-based store has a wide selection of contemporary
swimsuits, bras, and clothing. Sizes are listed according to
United Kingdom standards, but the Web site includes a conversion chart. Prices are converted upon purchase.
http://www.nicolajane.com

Notti™

This Canadian store sells different products that can cover
lumpectomy and mastectomy scars as well as abdominal scars.
The products come in a variety of colors and materials. They
also supply lingerie.
http://www.nottiwear.com

The Woman's Personal Health Resource, Inc.®
This business carries front-closure, compression, sports, leisure, and gel bras as well as swimwear, back supports, and other mastectomy products.
http://www.womanspersonalhealth.com
(877) 463-1343

Your Mind and Cancer Survivorship

Depression

National Mental Health Association
http://www.nmha.org
(703) 684-7722

Women's Health Experience™
http://www.womenshealthexperience.com
(513) 272-2198

Fertility Concerns and Female Cancer Survivors

American Academy of Adoption Attorneys
http://www.adoptionattorneys.org
(202) 832-2222

American Fertility Association
http://www.theafa.org
(888) 917-3777

Fertile Hope
http://www.fertilehope.org
(212) 242-6798

International Council on Infertility Information Dissemination (INCIID)
http://www.inciid.org
(703) 379 9178

Appendix

RESOLVE: The National Infertility Association
http://www.resolve.org
(888) 623-0744

Melissa Brisman Esq.
New Jersey
Attorney specializing in reproductive law.

Cancer centers offering fertility preservation surgery and other reproductive-sparing procedures

The Cornell Institute for Reproductive Medicine
Weill Medical College of Cornell University
505 East 70th Street, Suite 340
New York, NY 10021
(212) 746-1892
http://www.ivf.org

Memorial Sloan Kettering Cancer Center
1275 York Avenue
New York, NY 10021
(212) 639-2000
http://www.mskcc.org

The University of Texas M. D. Anderson Cancer Center
1515 Holcombe Boulevard
Houston, TX 77030
(800) 392-1611 or (713) 792-6161
http://www.mdanderson.org

Publications

Couples Confronting Cancer: Keeping Your Relationship Strong
by Katherine V. Bruss and Joy L. Fincannon
The American Cancer Society
(800) ACS-2345

Facing Forward: A Guide for Cancer Survivors
This National Cancer Institute publication has helpful sugges-
    tions and resources of how you can support other survivors in
    your area. The documents are now available on the Internet.
http://www.cancer.gov/cancerinfo/make-a-difference
(800) 4-CANCER

Sexual Health and Cancer Survivorship

Eve's Garden
Specializing in products to enhance women's sexuality.
http://www.evesgarden.com
(800) 848-3837

Female Sexual Dysfunction Online
Baylor College of Medicine and University of Medicine and
    Dentistry of New Jersey
http://www.femalesexualdysfunctiononline.org

National Vulvodynia Association (USA)
An online resource for patient support and education.
http://www.nva.org
(301) 299-0775

The American Association of Sexuality Educators, Counselors and Therapists
http://www.aasect.org
(804) 752-0026

Organizations

International Society for the Study of Women's Sexual Health
http://www.isswsh.org
(847) 517-7225

International Society of Sexuality and Cancer
http://www.issc.nt

The Alexander Foundation for Women's Health
Provides education for patients and clinicians on women's health
and gynecological psychiatry.
http://www.afwh.org
(510) 527-3010

The Women's Sexual Health Foundation
An educational resource about sexual health issues for patients
and clinicians.
http://www.twshf.org

Medications

Read the insert information that comes in the same package as
your medication. Ingredients as well as side effects are included.
More information is on the manufacturer's Web site.

http://www.arginimax.com
http://www.avlimil.com
http://www.viacreme-viacream-viagra.com
http://www.zestraforwomen.com

Glossary

Acoustic neuromas: Small, rare, slow-growing tumors that grow from the acoustic nerve (the nerve that is important for hearing).

Acupuncture: An ancient traditional Chinese medicine technique of inserting thin needles into the body at specific locations with the goal of restoring the normal flow of energy in the body. Often it is used to treat pain or other symptoms. This technique may help stimulate the nervous system, which releases brain hormones and transmitters. Acupuncture has been shown to help control hot flashes.

Analgesics: Type of medication used to treat pain.

Anemia: A condition in which the number of red blood cells is below normal.

Anticoagulant: A type of medication or substance (as a drug) that slows or stops fluid from clumping, especially coagulation of the blood. Also known as a blood thinner.

Antidepressant: A type of medication used to decrease the symptoms of low mood (depression).

Antiperspirant: A cosmetic preparation used in the underarm area that controls excessive perspiration and odor.

Aromatherapy: The ancient art of inhaling or using specific scents or aromas to help maintain bodily health. Essential oils can be inhaled to promote a quiet sense of peace.

Asbestos: A fibrous silicate material formerly used in thermal insulation, floor tiles, textiles, and was valued for its strength and endurance in many other products. Studies have linked asbestos dust to the development of cancer.

Benign: A type of non-cancerous tumor that can grow and press on surrounding structures, but does not invade surrounding structures or spread to a distant site.

Benzene: A colorless, flammable liquid with a sweet odor formed from natural processes like forest fires; also found in cigarette and cigar smoke and is used in dry cleaning fabrics.

Biopsy: A small amount of tissue removed during surgery or a less invasive procedure for later analysis by a pathologist.

Botanicals: Plants or plant parts valued for their medicinal properties; includes herbal products that are commonly prepared as a tea, an extract, or a tincture.

Breast self-examination (BSE): The act of examining your own breasts on a monthly basis to detect any changes. BSE should be preformed in a variety of positions including standing, sitting, and lying down. Visual inspection of the breasts should also occur.

Caffeine: A naturally occurring substance found in coffee and tea, most soft drinks (sodas), and many energy drinks. This substance can be added to medications for headaches. It acts as a nervous system stimulant and can increase mental alertness and wakefulness.

Cardiologist: A degreed and certified physician who specializes in the study of the heart and its action and diseases.

Chemotherapy: Treatment used after a tumor has been removed surgically to destroy any remaining cancer cells.

Chillow: A personal cooling pillow that may help with sleep. It works by keeping your head cool.

Colon: The large intestine, which is part of your gastrointestinal tract. Its function is to absorb water and food and to excrete stool.

Colonoscopy: A medical outpatient surgical procedure that is the screening tool to detect colonic abnormalities and precancerous growths in the colon.

Colposcopy: A procedure that uses a specialized machine called a colposcope, which is a magnifying instrument designed to facilitate visual inspection of the vagina and cervix. Women with abnormal cells on their Pap test may be required to undergo this outpatient procedure to visualize and possibly sample (biopsy) the cervical tissues.

Compliance: The process of following a regimen of treatment; the act of taking and following prescribed medications and or instructions given by your healthcare provider.

Computed tomography (CT scan): A highly sensitive radiology imaging technique used to help diagnose a disease; used periodically to check the progress of tumors in patients with cancer.

Consent form: A written document signed by a patient to indicate that someone (most likely their physician) has explained to the patient about a particular treatment, including its risks and benefits; signing the form means that the patient agrees to receive the treatment; also referred to as "informed consent."

Dowager's hump: An abnormal outward curvature of the upper back; round shoulders and spinal changes result in an abnormally stooped posture. This can be caused especially by bone loss and compression of the vertebrae, which commonly occurs in osteoporosis.

Dyspareunia: Pain or discomfort during sexual intercourse.

Endocrinologist: A degreed, certified physician who specializes in diagnosing and treating hormone disorders.

Endometrial biopsy: An office-based procedure where a small plastic instrument called a pipelle is placed within the uterus and a small sample of uterine or endometrial tissue is obtained.

Estrogen: A female hormone produced by the ovaries; it is responsible for female changes during maturity.

Female androgen insufficiency: A syndrome characterized by blunted or diminished motivation, persistent fatigue, and a decreased sense of personal well being that may be characterized by insufficient plasma estrogen, low circulating bioavailability testosterone, and low sexual desire (libido).

Guided imagery: A technique in which patients use their imagination to dream something they desire (e.g., visualizing the chemotherapy attacking their cancer cells; sometimes used during therapy as a relaxation strategy; many tapes and CDs are available with music and voice scripted for a specific guided journey).

Gynecological oncologist: A degreed, certified physician specializing in the treatment of cancer of the female reproductive system.

Hair transplantation: A surgical procedure that moves hair follicles from one area to another to help lessen thinning hair, particularly on the crown of the head.

Hormone replacement therapy (HRT): Estrogen and progesterone that can be given in various combinations to relieve the symptoms of menopause. When estrogen is given alone it is called estrogen replacement.

Hypersomnia: Sleeping all of the time.

Hypertension (also known as high blood pressure): An abnormally high arterial blood pressure that typically results from a thickening of blood vessel walls; a risk factor for various illnesses such as heart attack, heart failure, stroke, or end-stage renal (kidney) disease.

Hypnosis: A technique used to induce a trancelike state that consists of altered consciousness. It is also known to resemble sleep but it is typically induced by a person/hypnotist whose suggestions can be readily accepted by the subject.

Immunosuppression: When the body's natural immune responses are lowered by drugs or an illness; this condition increases the body's susceptibility to infection.

Infertility: An inability to begin (conceive) or complete a pregnancy for the entire nine months (gestation). In more simple terms, a woman is no longer able to become pregnant because her ovaries are no longer producing reproductive hormones like estrogen or progesterone that can mature an egg, or her uterus is unable to hold or maintain the fetus for the duration of a pregnancy.

Insomnia: Lack of sleep.

Kegel exercises: Exercises designed to increase muscle strength and elasticity in the pelvis; often recommended for the treatment of urinary incontinence.

Laparoscopy: Camera-directed surgery done without creating a large incision into the abdomen.

Laughter therapy: A type of treatment based in the premise that the patient gains physical and mental benefits from laughter, including lowered blood pressure, decreased anxiety and stress hormones, release of endorphins (the body's natural pain killers), and a general sense of well-being.

Lead: Commonly found in household items. When inhaled or ingested may cause many ill effects.

Letrozole: An anti-estrogen type of medication.

Lumpectomy: Excision of a breast tumor with a limited amount of associated tissue.

Magnetic resonance imaging (MRI scan): A diagnostic test that creates images of structures in the body using radio waves and a powerful magnet.

Malignant: A type of cancerous tumor that can invade surrounding structures and spread to a distant site in the body; even if treated, malignant tumors may cause death.

Mammography: A special X-ray imaging of the breast where the radiation exposure of the breast tissue is minimal.

Meditation: Ancient techniques using deep, slow breathing to calm the mind and help the body relax; often used in conjunction with visualization.

Menopause: Physical changes marking the end of a woman's fertile years, the most notable being the cessation of the menstrual cycles.

Menstruation: Vaginal bleeding due to endometrial shedding following ovulation when the egg is not fertilized.

Music therapy: A therapeutic technique exposing the patient to the pleasures of music, either by listening or playing an instrument, in the company of a psychotherapist specializing in this technique. Creativity, inner peace, and personal pleasure can be enhanced while self-expression can promote an improved sense of well being.

Obesity: The medical condition referring to a severely overweight patient.

Obstetrician: A degreed, certified physician specializing in the care of a woman and her offspring during her pregnancy, childbirth, and shortly after her delivery.

Oncologist: A degreed, certified physician who specializes in treating cancer. Surgical oncologists specialize in cancer surgery; medical oncologists specialize in treatment with chemotherapy, hormonal therapy, and biological therapy; radiation oncologists specialize in treatments with radiation.

Osteoporosis: A condition that is characterized by a decrease in bone mass and density (thinning of the bones), causing bones to become fragile.

Ovulation: Process of egg release from the ovary.

Pacemaker: An electrical device that is surgically implanted into the chest that is used for stimulating or steadying the heartbeat.

Pap test: A type of medical test used for the early detection of cancer, especially of the cervix; involves sampling cells and staining them by a special technique that differentiates diseased tissue from normal tissue; also called *Papanicolaou smear*, *Papanicolaou test*, and *Pap smear*.

Pedometer: A small device that can measure your steps, calories burned, and distance that you have walked or jogged.

Pet therapy: A therapeutic strategy that helps a patient get involved with a dog, cat, or other type of pet; enjoying time and leisure activities with the pet helps the patient's general health.

Phantom pain: A type of painful sensation that can occur at the site of an amputation or limb removal; some women who have had mastectomies or complete breast removal can feel abnormal pain, sensations, or discomfort at the area where the breast is missing.

Polyp: A projecting mass of swollen tissue that may appear in the intestine or on the cervix. Endometrial polyps occur within the uterine cavity. Most are benign.

Positron emission tomography (PET scan): A specialized imaging test used for diagnosis that can see inside sections of the body.

Prophylactic mastectomy: When normal breast tissue is removed in the unaffected breast to help minimize the risk of recurrence or the development of another new primary breast cancer.

Prophylactic oophorectomy (risk-reducing bilateral salpingo-oophorectomy, RRBSO): Removal of a woman's eggs and ovaries in an attempt to reduce or eliminate a risk for future cancer.

Psychiatrist: A degreed, credentialed physician who specializes in the prevention, diagnosis, and treatment of mental illness; a psychiatrist can prescribe medicine.

Psychologist: A degreed, credentialed therapist who councils with patients and their families about emotional and personal matters and can help them make ethical decisions.

Reflexology: A type of alternative therapy using massage and pressure applied to the foot to relieve stress, pain, and promote circulation.

Reiki: A technique of hands-on touching based on the belief that this touching channels the body's spiritual energy and leads to spiritual and physical healing.

Remission: Subsiding of disease; the disease is still present but either it is undetectable to the patient or it has no symptoms.

Shiatsu: A type of massage involving pressure and bodily stretching to maintain optimum health; Swedish massage relieves tension by deeply kneading muscles.

Sodoku: A type of number puzzle with a 9 × 9 grid subdivided into nine 3 × 3 grids with scattered clues.

Tantra: Ancient Indian spiritual tradition and belief system with the premise that sexuality is tied into personal energy and is capable of changing us if we submit to our primal sexual desires while maintaining control and heightening spiritual awareness. When incorporated into lovemaking, tantra ultimately intensifies the sexual dynamic or consciousness between couples.

Tetrachlorethylene: A toxic agent commercially produced for the dry cleaning industry and textile business.

Total hysterectomy: Surgical removal of the uterus and cervix.

Translucent: A type of barrier that diffuses the passage of light.

Transvaginal ultrasound: An imaging technique using high frequency sound waves; a probe is placed in the vagina to assess the female pelvic anatomy.

Tubal ligation: The destruction or ligation (tying) of the fallopian tubes to prevent passage of the egg or ova from the ovaries into the uterus; a method of female sterilization or contraception.

Tubal pregnancy: A type of pregnancy where the egg has implanted in the fallopian tube instead of the uterus. This can be a serious medical condition and needs immediate medical attention.

Tumor: A mass of cells or tissue that grows abnormally.

Vaginal atrophy: When the vaginal tissues decrease in size, become pale or dry without lubrication; this is usually a result of decreased hormones in the woman's body (as in menopause or other medical conditions) which affects these sensitive tissues.

Yoga: A type of exercise where the emphasis is on long, slow stretching into various postures and using slow, deep breathing to hold the posture. It is said to unify the elements of mind and body to help eliminate stress and decrease fatigue.

Index

gender and genetics, 19
  medical conditions, 19
Ovarian cancer, 34–37
  incidence, 35
  risk factors, 35–36
    increased risk population, 35
  screening for
    blood testing, 36
    pelvic examinations, 36
    transvaginal ultrasound, 36–37
  symptoms, 35
  talcum powder associated with, 60
Ovarian shielding or ovarian transposition, 190
Ovarian tissue freezing and transplantation, 189–190
Ovulation, defined, 186, 245
Oz, Mehmet, 78

P

Pacemaker
  defined, 245
  effects of cell phone use on, 61
PAHs (polycyclic aromatic hydrocarbons), 64–65
Pain management, 103–112
  fears about pain medication addiction, 104
  medications
    antidepressants or anticonvulsants, 107
    delaying treatment with, 107–108
    non-opioids, 106–107
    opioids, 107
    questions to ask your physician before taking, 105–106
  non-medication ways to control pain, 108
  phantom pain, 104
  professionals who can help you, 103
  sexual dysfunction, 210–211
  treatment, 104–105
  web site, 235
Pap test, 25–29
  categories of results
    AGUS (atypical glandular cells of undetermined significance), 28
    ASCUS (atypical cells of undetermined significance), 27–28
    normal, 27
    squamous intraepithelial lesions, 28
  defined, 14, 245
  description of, 27
  follow-up and compliance, 28

frequency of, guidelines for, 26–27
  human papilloma virus (HPV), 28–29
  importance of the test, 25
  informational web sites, 234
Paroxetine, for hot flashes, 125
Paxil, for hot flashes, 125
Pedigree, genetic testing, 37–38
Pedometer
  defined, 24, 245
  using a pedometer, 90
Pelvic cancer, associated with diethylstilbestrol (DES), 62–63
People Living with Cancer, web site, 232
PET scan (positron emission tomography), defined, 2, 245
Pet therapy, 159–160
  defined, 159, 245
Phantom pain, defined, 104, 245
Phosphodiesterase inhibitors, 207, 216–217
Photoaging, 54
Physical examination, 13
Pocket Rocket, The, 222
Polycyclic aromatic hydrocarbons (PAHs), 64–65
Polyp
  defined, 49, 245
  removal of, 49
Positron emission tomography (PET scan), defined, 2, 245
"Predictors of Adoption Maintenance of Vigorous Physical Activity in Men and Women," 94
Pregnancy. See also Fertility
  natural, after cancer treatment, 190–191
  and reduced risk of certain cancers, 32, 36
Premarin, 131, 213
Premature ovarian failure, 184
Prevention of cancer. See specific types of cancer
Progestin/progesterone therapy, 115–116, 132–133
Propecia treatment, for hair loss, 145
Prophylactic mastectomy
  defined, 39, 245
  described, 39–40
Prophylactic oophorectomy (risk reducing oophorectomy RRBSO)
  defined, 245
  negative sexual consequences from, 202–203
Protein, 71
Psychiatrist, defined, 245